ATLAS OF
CONGENITAL CARDIAC DISEASE

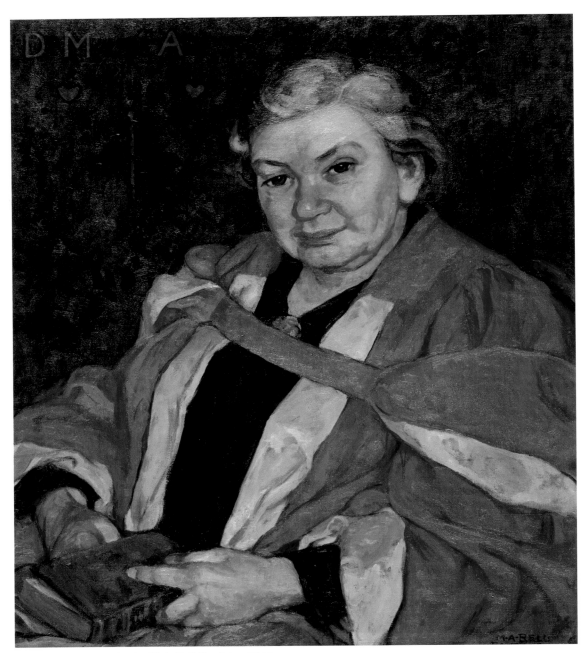

Maude Abbott, painting by M.A. Bell Eastlake, 1940

ATLAS
OF
CONGENITAL CARDIAC
DISEASE

MAUDE E. ABBOTT

With an Introduction by Richard Fraser

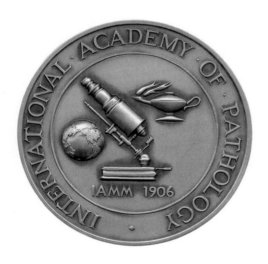

Published in Commemoration
of the
100th Anniversary of the Founding
of the International Academy of Pathology

MᴄGILL-QUEEN'S UNIVERSITY PRESS
Montreal & Kingston • London • Ithaca

© McGill-Queen's University Press 2006

ISBN-13: 978-0-7735-3128-4   ISBN-10: 0-7735-3128-9

Legal deposit third quarter 2006
Bibliothèque nationale du Québec

Printed in Canada on acid-free paper that is 100% ancient forest free
(100% post-consumer recycled), processed chlorine free.

McGill-Queen's University Press acknowledges the support of the Canada Council for
the Arts for our publishing program. We also acknowledge the financial support of
the Government of Canada through the Book Publishing Industry Development
Program (BPIDP) for our publishing activities.

Library and Archives Canada Cataloguing in Publication

Abbott, Maude E. (Maude Elizabeth), 1869-1940
Atlas of congenital cardiac disease / Maude E. Abbott ; with an introduction by
Richard Fraser. – New ed.

Includes index.

ISBN-13: 978-0-7735-3128-4   ISBN-10: 0-7735-3128-9

1. Congenital heart disease—Atlases. I. International Academy of Pathology
II. Title.

RC687.A33 2006   616.1'20430222   C2006-901739-5

CONTENTS

ACKNOWLEDGMENTS

The digital photography of the Abbott specimens and the electronic remastering of the images were carried out by Kamilah Roberts-McIntosh and Leena Narsinghani, both of the McGill University Pathology Department. Their good spirits and dedication were outstanding and they were both a joy to work with. Pamela Miller and Chistopher Lyons of the Osler Library, McGill University, provided invaluable assistance in research as well as access to documents and the London Exhibit posters. I would also like to thank Dr Fred Silva, executive director of the International Academy of Pathology, Dr Bill Gardner, director of the American Registry of Pathology, Dr Abe Fuks, dean of the McGill Faculty of Medicine, and Philip Cercone, chief editor at McGill-Queens University Press, for their encouragement and support. Susanne McAdam and Joan McGilvray, also of McGill-Queen's University Press, provided able assistance in production and editing. The members of the Abbott family, particularly Kim and Elizabeth, were involved at several points in discussions of the re-publication and their input is also appreciated.

Finally, generous grants without which the project would not have been able to proceed were received from Abbott Canada Inc., Associated Medical Services, and Caprion Pharmaceuticals Inc.

INTRODUCTION
Maude Abbott
and the
Atlas of Congenital Cardiac Disease

Maude Abbott is one of the best known Canadian physicians of the twentieth century.[1] Born in 1869 in St Andrew's East, a small town in Quebec, she was raised by her grandmother, her father having abandoned the family shortly before her birth and her mother having died shortly after it. In her senior year of high school she won a scholarship to McGill University, from which she obtained a bachelor's degree in Arts in 1890. After being refused entry to the McGill Medical School, which did not accept women, she attended Bishop's College, a relatively small institution with a medical school in Montreal. She received her medical degree in 1894, taking the Senior Prize in anatomy and the Chancellor's Prize for the best examination in the final sessions.

Following postgraduate studies in Europe in pathology and internal medicine, she returned to Montreal in 1897 to establish a private practice. Soon thereafter she was introduced to George Adami, chair of Pathology at McGill, who urged her to investigate and publish on a case of hemochromatosis. Her work on this and other projects so impressed Adami that he appointed her assistant curator of the Medical Museum in 1898. The museum curatorship — which she took over completely in 1901 — proved to be the central point of her academic life. Her work in the development and cataloging of its collection led to demonstrations of specimens for students which were so well received that they became a compulsory part of the pathology course in 1904. She was also a co-founder of the International Association of Medical Museums in 1906 and secretary-treasurer of the organization until her death in 1940. Finally, museum activities led directly to her study of congenital heart disease, which culminated in the 1936 *Atlas* reprinted here.

Abbott was actively involved in the McGill Medical Museum until 1923, when she left Montreal to take up the position of Acting Chair of Pathology at the Woman's Medical College of Pennsylvania. She returned to McGill in 1925 as assistant professor of Medicine. This brief period away from "home" was a reflection of the difficulties she had with the McGill administration throughout her career — she never received an academic rank higher than assistant professor and was effectively relieved from museum teaching in 1923. Despite this, she became well known and respected throughout the world as a proponent of the International Association of Medical Museums and editor of its bulletin, and as an investigator of cardiac anomalies, on which subject she published numerous case reports and reviews. She also developed an interest in history, publish-

ing articles and books on subjects related to the McGill Medical Faculty, the city of Montreal, Quebec medicine, and nursing. She was active in the development of the Canadian War Museum, the McGill Medical History Museum, and the Argenteuil Museum of local history, near her birthplace. She succeeded in all these endeavors while taking care of her sister, who suffered for many years from manic-depressive illness. Abbott retired from McGill in 1936, but continued her academic interests and was planning to write a textbook on congenital cardiovascular disease at the time of her death in 1940.

When Abbott published her *Atlas of Congenital Cardiac Disease* in 1936,[2] it represented the culmination of over thirty-five years of work. Her involvement in what was at the time a relatively obscure aspect of medicine was profoundly influenced by two chance occurrences in 1899 — her "discovery" of the Holmes heart and a meeting with William Osler in Baltimore. At the end of the nineteenth century the McGill Medical Museum was in a state of disarray. When Osler moved to Philadelphia in 1884, he left McGill an impressive collection of autopsy specimens; however, this collection and material donated to the museum in the years before Osler were poorly organized and seldom used in teaching. In an attempt to bring some order to the collection, the job of museum curator was included in the responsibilities of the chair of Pathology when it was established by the Faculty of Medicine in 1892. The first chair, George Adami, did little with the collection other than add to it. He appointed Abbott assistant curator in 1898 and suggested that she visit museums at teaching centers in the United States to learn how they were organized. During this trip she met Osler, who told her:

I wonder, now, if you realize what an opportunity *you* have? That McGill Museum is a great place. As soon as you go home look up the *British Medical Journal* for 1893, and read the article by Mr. Jonathan Hutchinson on "A Clinical Museum." That is what he calls his museum in London and it is the greatest place I know for teaching students in. Pictures of life and death together. Wonderful. You read it and see what *you* can do.[3]

Abbott took these words to heart and upon her return to Montreal in early 1899 began working on the museum in earnest, reviewing, cataloging, and classifying specimens in the collection. Shortly thereafter she found an unusual heart labeled "ulcerative endocarditis." Unable to find any additional clinical or pathological information on the specimen, she wrote to Osler, who informed her that the heart had been given to McGill in 1822 by Andrew Holmes, one of the four founders of the McGill Medical School and the first dean of its Medical Faculty. The case history and pathologic description of the heart had been reported by Holmes in the *Transactions of the Medico-chirurgical Society of Edinburgh* in 1824 (Fig. 1A). Abbott republished the case in the *Montreal Medical Journal* in 1901 (Fig. 1B), expanding the morphological discussion and adding a historical review. This work was an important beginning to her life-long interest in congenital cardiovascular disease.

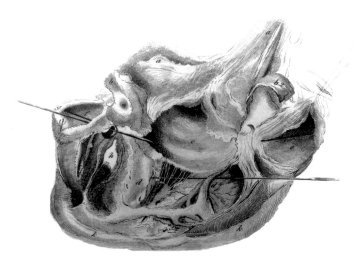

Fig. 1 A. Drawing of the Holmes heart, from Holmes' article in the *Transactions of the Edinburgh Medico-chirurgical Society*, 1824.
B. Diagnostic sketch of the Holmes heart by R. Tait Mackenzie, from Abbott's article in the *Montreal Medical Journal*, July 1901

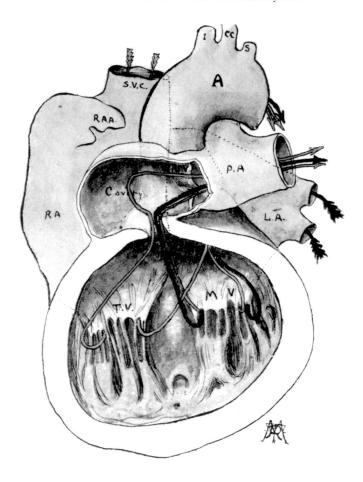

Abbott's plan for the Medical Museum as a whole was to group specimens according to what she called the "Osler, or Descriptive, Catalogue," in which material displayed in the museum was to be organized according to organ system and associated with clinical information provided by physicians knowledgeable on the subject. Specimen descriptions and corresponding case histories and medical discussions were to be published in a series of books that students could use as a guide for study in the museum. Osler helped raise money for this project and the first volume, on the hematopoietic system, was published in 1915.[4] Abbott had been working on the catalogue of the circulatory system long before this and had sent a draft of the endocardial section to Osler in 1905. He was clearly impressed with the work, writing to tell her "what a splendid section it is," and invited her to contribute a chapter on congenital heart disease to his 1908 edition of the *The Principles and Practice of Medicine*. Following Olser's advice to treat the subject "statistically," she undertook a review of the literature. Beginning with the *Transactions of the Pathological Society of London*, she summarized all the clinical and pathological information related to cardiac anomalies available in the medical journals of the day, eventually documenting 412 cases. She continued to add to this list over the years, listing over 1,000 cases in a chart in the 1936 *Atlas*.

Abbott continued to collect specimens illustrating cardiovascular anomalies, many from McGill teaching hospitals and some from colleagues around the world. In 1931 she organized a series of diagrams, photographs, and drawings of pathologic specimens and the clinical material associated with them for display at the Graduate Fortnight in Cardiology hosted by the New York Academy of Medicine. The following year she sent much of this material and some of the corresponding museum specimens as an exhibit to the Centenary Meeting of the British Medical Association in London, England (Fig. 2). The graphic material for the exhibit was displayed on a series of millboard posters (Plates 1, 2, and 3) which, when arranged for display, occupied a wall space about four feet high by thirty-two feet long. Approximately fifty anatomical specimens were included in the exhibit on two tiers of shelving below the posters. The exhibit was organized in two sections, one on development and comparative anatomy of the heart and the other on cases, diagrams, and illustrations of a variety of cardiac abnormalities (in a section titled "Clinical Classification of Congenital Cardiac Disease"). Cases in the second section were in turn arranged in three groups — cardiac anomalies with no abnormal systemic-pulmonary connection, cases associated with an arteriovenous shunt, and cases with a permanent venous-arterial shunt. The exhibit appears to have been a success and was re-presented at a joint meeting of the American and Canadian Medical Associations in Atlantic City in 1935 and at a meeting of the Ontario Medical Association in 1936. Abbott described the London exhibit in the British Medical Journal:

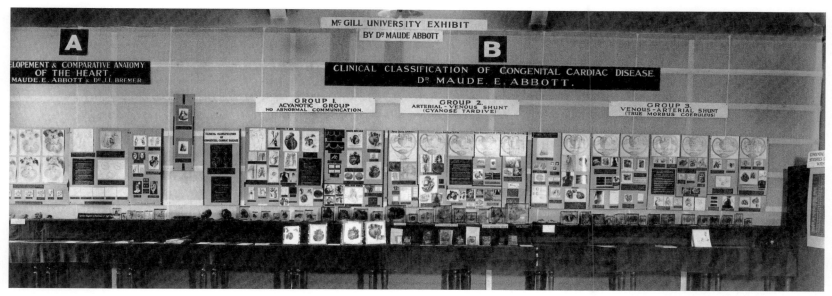

Fig. 2 Photograph of the 1932 London exhibit.

The artistic merit of the many fine medical art drawings interpolated in the wall display, and the skillful technique manifested in the mounting and stencil labeling of the specimens, made this exhibit one of the most attractive parts of the museum. Its chief value, and its really exceptional interest, however, lay not so much in these features, or in the scientific and historical importance of the many unique cases portrayed, as in the fact that this collection, representing as it did the fruits of many years of investigation, revealed the expansion from a relatively small nucleus of original observations of an ordered whole, and told a coherent story in which were made apparent the etiologic basis of congenital cardiac disease and the clinical significance of the various groups into which antenatal lesions fall.[5]

Following Abbott's return from London in 1932, Dr David Seecof of the Jewish General Hospital in Montreal suggested that the exhibit material might form the basis for an atlas; Abbott quickly agreed. Her original idea was to reproduce the exhibit exactly as it had appeared in London and a dummy atlas was prepared on this basis. However, in this format the diagrams had to be very small and it was decided to dissemble the material from the London Exhibit posters, add additional cases, and re-organize the material in a series of twenty-five plates that included diagrams and photographs of both gross and microscopic cardiac anomalies as well as associated clinical material such as electrocardiograph tracings, radiographs, and patient photographs. Detailed descriptions of case histories and the specific features of individual specimens or diseases accompanied the plates.

The *Atlas* was published by the American Heart Association in 1936. The members of the executive committee of this organization supported the project cautiously, indicating to Abbott that "the expenses of publishing and distribution are to be met out of the proceeds of the sale, supplemented if necessary by funds advanced by you."[6] The list price was $5.50. As it turned out, Abbott arranged

enough advance subscriptions to "come out of the undertaking solvent from the sale of the first 750 copies."[7] She proceeded to have an additional 250 copies bound in the hope of making a profit. The *Atlas* was also a critical success. A reviewer writing in the *American Heart Journal* in 1937 said:

In this Atlas, Dr. Abbott has epitomized her monumental knowledge of congenital cardiac disease and has presented it clearly and simply in the combination of text and superb illustrations. The book is recommended to all with any interest in the subject of heart disease and should be in the library of the general practitioner as well as the specialist. It is destined to become a medical classic."[8]

A second printing was undertaken in 1954, prompted by "numerous requests" to the Heart Association for additional copies. In a review of this printing in 1955, Dr. James Watt stated:

With the ... development of physiological methods for study and surgical techniques for the treatment of these congenital defects, current knowledge extends far beyond that contained in this monograph. However, it represented one of the most important contributions to the knowledge of these defects and continues to stand as a monument to Dr. Abbott, who contributed so much and helped provide the stimulus for the rapid advances in the diagnostic, physiologic, and surgical aspects of congenital heart disease over the past two decades.[9]

A second reviewer writing in the *American Heart Journal* at the same time stated:

For the younger student of congenital heart disease [the *Atlas*] will supply the historic background to give him a well balanced outlook on modern advances ... For the older student of cardiac anomalies this still stands as a valuable reference book, often referred to. Even yet it amazes the reviewer to find illustrative cases, descriptions of which are difficult to discover in the literature.[10]

As these testimonials suggest, Abbott's work, as exemplified in the *Atlas*, laid the groundwork for understanding the morphology and pathogenesis of congenital cardiac abnormalities and, ultimately, for their treatment in the latter part of the twentieth century. Abbott may have forseen some of these developments, since she had plans to follow the *Atlas* with a more extensive textbook. In a description of the planned book used in applications for publishing grants, she wrote:

The work proposed is a complete revision of our present knowledge of congenital cardiac disease, together with the accumulation of new data which will enable the applicant to draw more positive conclusions upon the clinical significance of the various types of cardiac defects, the value or otherwise of operative interference in the acyanotic cases and the attendant risks involved, the bearing of various physiologic processes upon the prognosis in such patients, as also the influence of heredity and ante-natal conditions in general upon the genesis of such lesions.[11]

Her plans for this work included a complete revision of the cases documented in the "statistical" chart included in the London exhibit and illustrated in the *Atlas*, with emphasis on prognosis ("duration of life"), the effects of pregnancy and lactation, the incidence of endocarditis and other complications, and the indications for surgical intervention. In 1940 she received a grant of $2,500 from the Carnegie Foundation for the project and planned to spend time in Boston and New York on research. According to an application to the Guggenheim Memorial Foundation at about the same time, she hoped to begin the project in January 1941 and complete it by September 1942. However in July 1940, before she could begin serious work, she suffered a cerebral hemorrhage, from which she eventually died in September of the same year

The exact number of specimens exemplifying congenital cardiovascular disease that remained in the McGill Medical Museum following Abbott's death in 1940 is unclear. However, in the mid-1940s approximately eighty were transferred from the Strathcona Medical Building (the site of Abbott's Medical Museum) to the pathology museum in the nearby Pathological Institute. In the 1960s the preservative fluid in the specimen jars was replaced and the collection was placed in a display cabinet in a newly built wing of the Institute. Digital images were made of the entire Abbott collection in 2003–04 and were subsequently enhanced by "removing" their glass cases as well as the accumulated sediment and debris within the preservative fluid. A selection of these images is included in

this memorial volume (Plates 4 to 22), using the specimen numbers given during restoration in the 1960s. Seventeen of the Abbott specimens specifically referred to in the *Atlas* are included.

The re-publication of the *Atlas* in 2006 coincides with the one hundredth anniversary of the founding of the International Association of Medical Museums. The concept of such an association originated in 1898 with Wyatt Johnson, who suggested to Abbott that she and the curator of the Army Medical Museum in Washington DC should organize "a society of curators." The idea was discussed on and off for a number of years and finally came to fruition in 1906 at a meeting in Washington of Abbott, James Carroll (of the Army Medical Museum), and John McCallum (of Johns Hopkins Hospital). Carroll was the first president of the Association and Abbott was the secretary-treasurer, a position that she held until her death in 1940.

Following the decline of the medical museum as a teaching aid in the middle of the twentieth century, accompanied by an increasing emphasis on experimental and diagnostic surgical pathology, the Association changed its name to the International Academy of Pathology in 1955. The Academy has since grown remarkably and at the time of this writing includes approximately 45 divisions around the world and a membership of over 17,000 pathologists. Republication of the *Atlas* is meant to serve as a testimony to a great physician as well as a memorial to the two most important legacies of her professional life — medical museums and the association she co-founded to promote their principles, and the study of congenital cardiovascular disease.

Notes

1 H. E. MacDermot, *Maude Abbott: A Memoir* (Toronto: MacMillan Press, 1941); D. Waugh, *Maudie of McGill: Dr. Maude Abbott and the Foundations of Heart Surgery* (Toronto: Hannah Institute and Dundurn Press, 1992)

2 M. Abbott, *Atlas of Congenital Cardiac Disease* (New York: The American Heart Association, 1936)

3 M. Abbott, "The pathological collections of the late Sir William Osler at McGill University," *Bulletin of the International Association of Medical Museums* 9 (1926): 185–99

4 O. Gruner, M., edited by M. Abbott, *Descriptive Catalogue of the Medical Museum of McGill University*. Part IV: Section "The Hematopoietic Organs" (Oxford: Oxford University Press, 1915).

5 M. Abbott, "The McGill University exhibit: Development of the heart and the clinical classification of congenital cardiac disease," *British Medical Journal* (31 Dec. 1932): 1197.

6 Letter from H.M. Marvin , chairman of the Executive Committee, American Heart Association, to Maude Abbott, 21 Nov. 1935, Osler Library, Abbott Box 249, 438/84.

7 M. Abbott, letter to Mrs. M.N. Kettle, 6 October 1936. Cited in MacDermot, *Maude Abbott*, 182-3.

8 Anonymous review, *American Heart Journal* 13 (1937): 254.

9 J. Watt, *Bulletin of the Medical Library Association* 43 (1955): 583–4.

10 Anonymous review, *American Heart Journal* 49 (1955): 938–9.

11 Maude Abbott, undated document, "Plans for Work," Osler Library, Abbott Box 249, 438/84.

COLOUR PLATES

PLATE I   POSTER "CONGENITAL CYANOSIS" FROM THE 1932 LONDON EXHIBIT

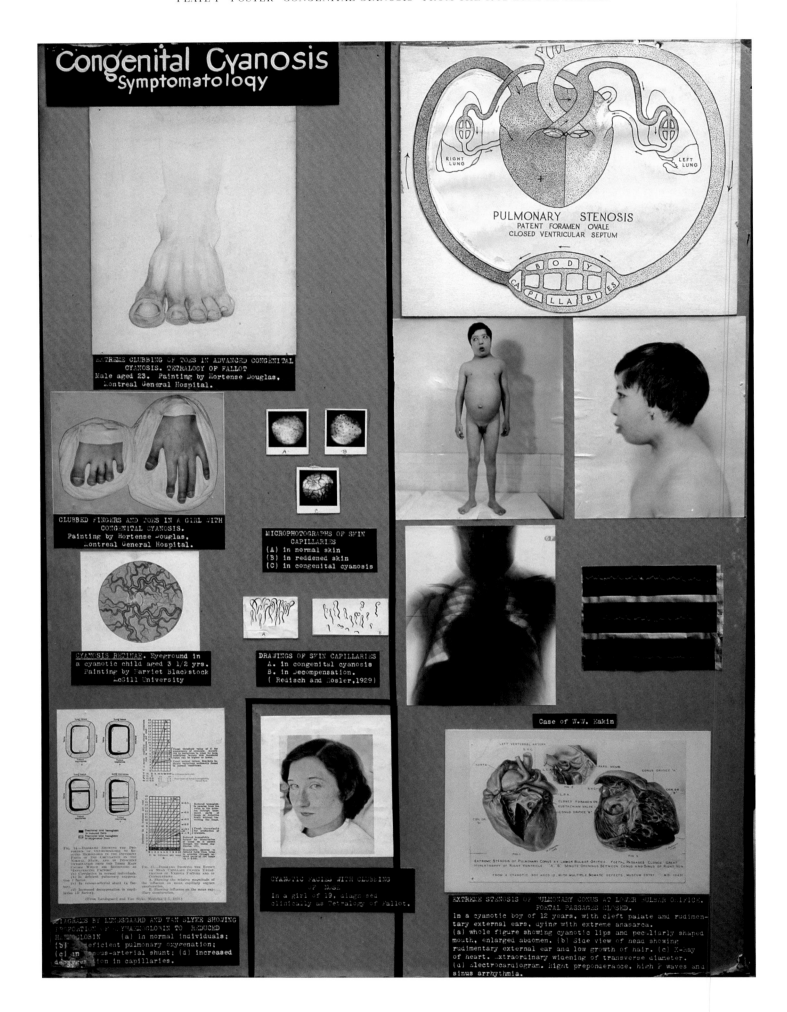

PLATE II   POSTER "BICUSPID AORTIC VALVE" FROM THE 1932 LONDON EXHIBIT

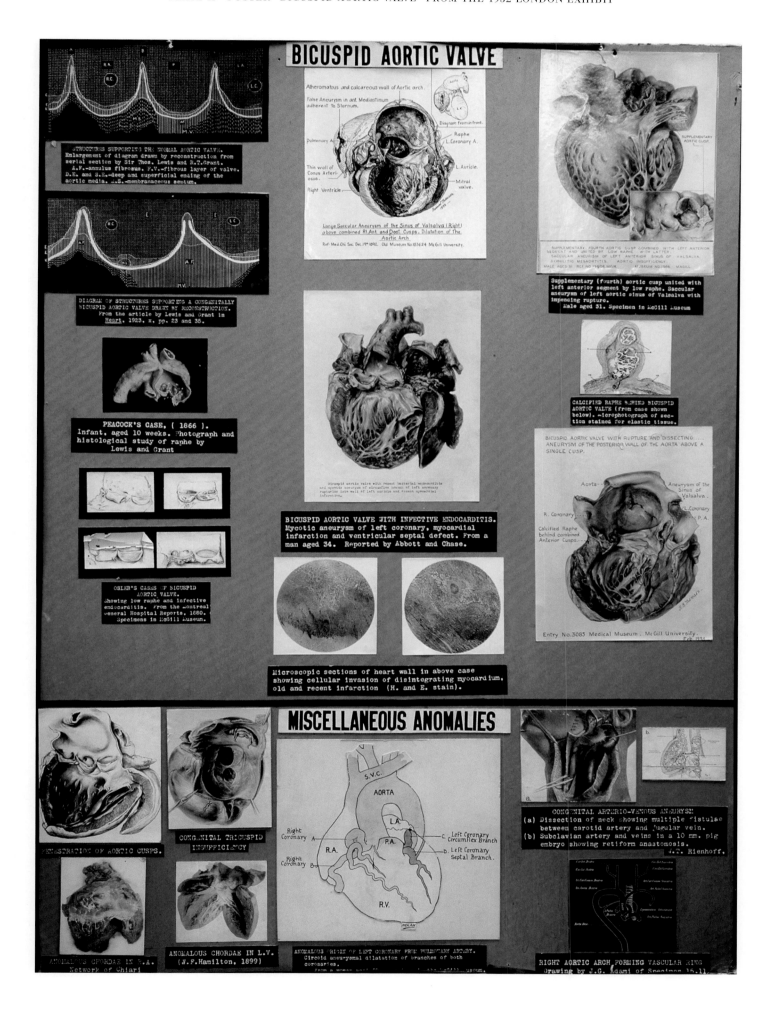

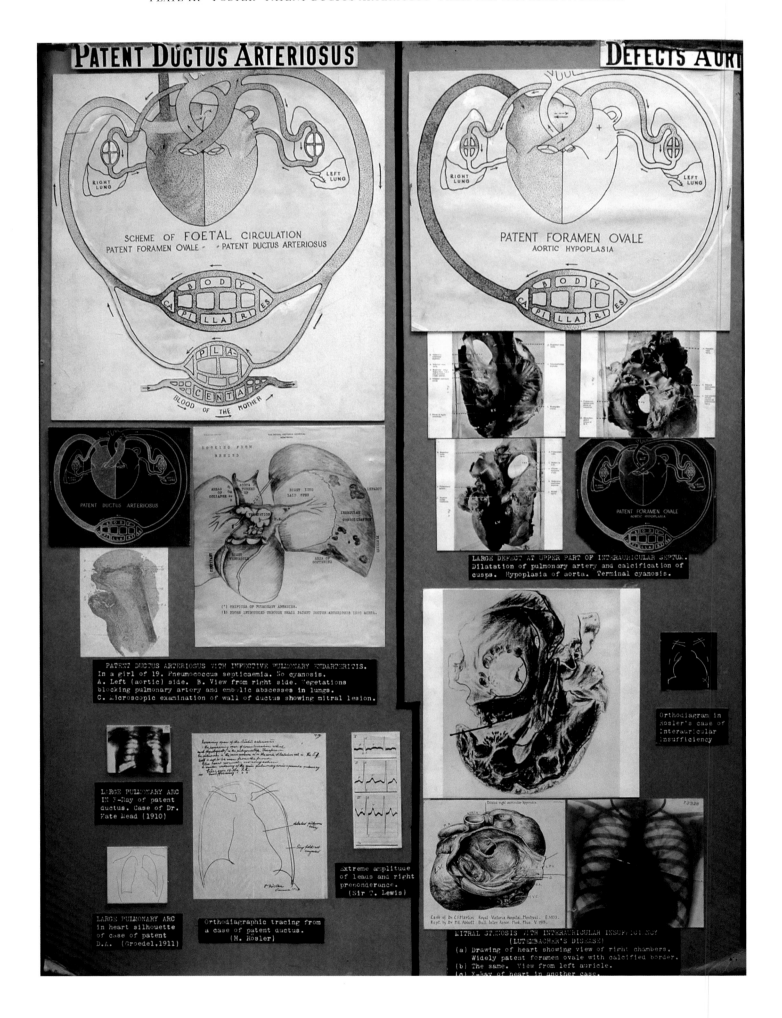

PLATE IV   FISH HEARTS

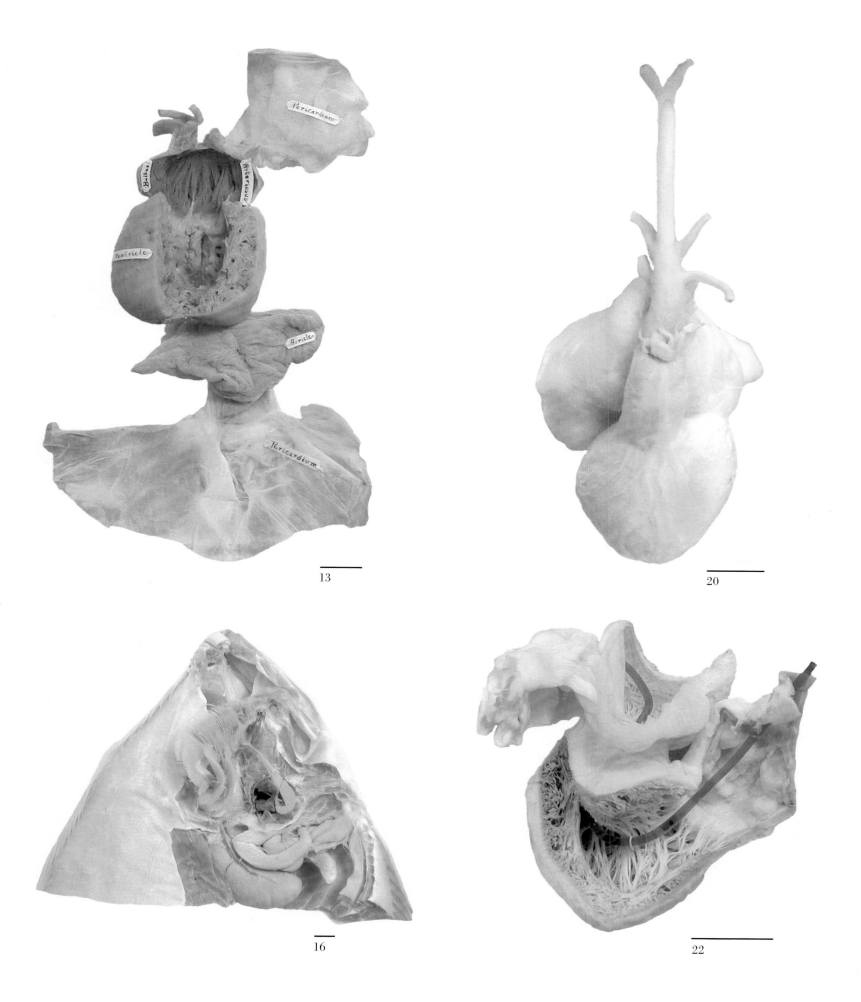

13

20

16

22

13 Heart of Angler (Lophius piscatorius). A large heart appearing externally two chambered. Arterial trunks from top; auricle below. *Atlas*, Plate II, Fig 1. 1918.

20 Heart of Shark. Ventral view showing conus arteriosus, bulbis cordis, common ventricle and auricle. Unknown date.

16 Heart of Flounder. 1919.

22 Heart of fish. Unknown date.

Specimen numbers are those given during restoration of the collection in the 1960s. Black bar indicates 1 cm.

PLATE V   FISH AND REPTILIAN HEARTS: CLINICAL CLASSIFICATION

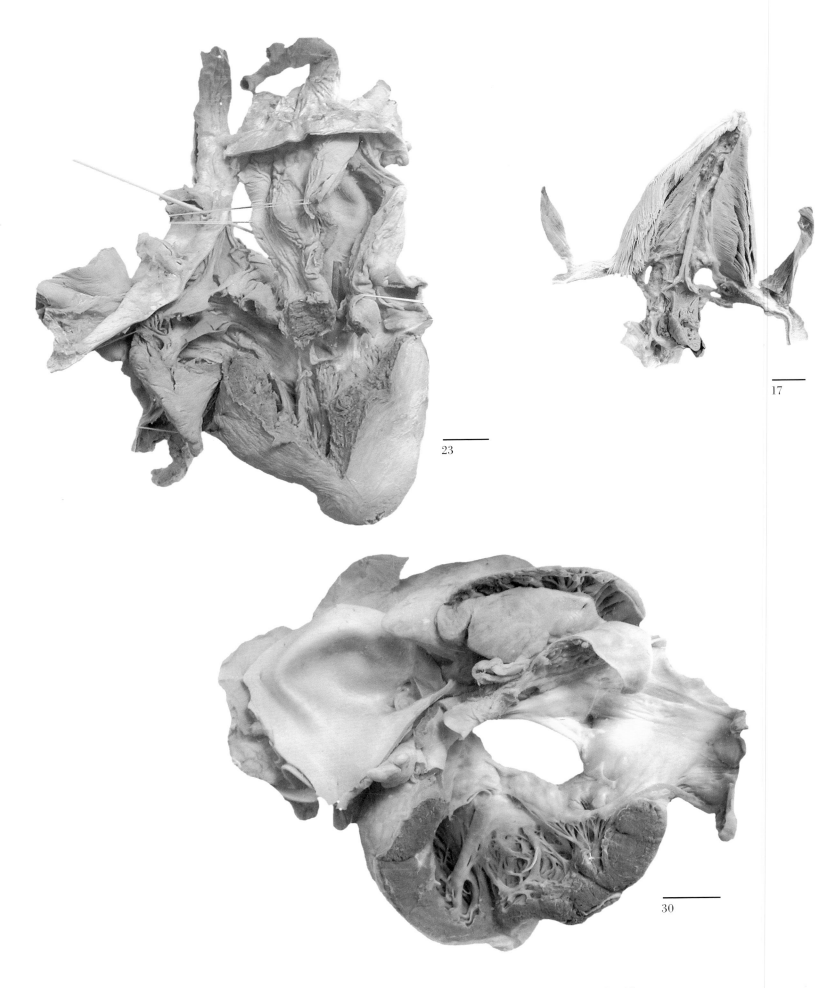

23

17

30

23 Heart of Alligator. Unknown date.

17 Heart of Eel. Mouth region and pectoral fins showing tubular bulbus arteriosus. 1919.

30 Persistent Ostium Primum. Double mitral orifice; bifid apex. Five-year-old girl. *Atlas*, Plate V, Fig 2b. 1907.

PLATE VI ANOMALIES OF THE AORTIC ARCH

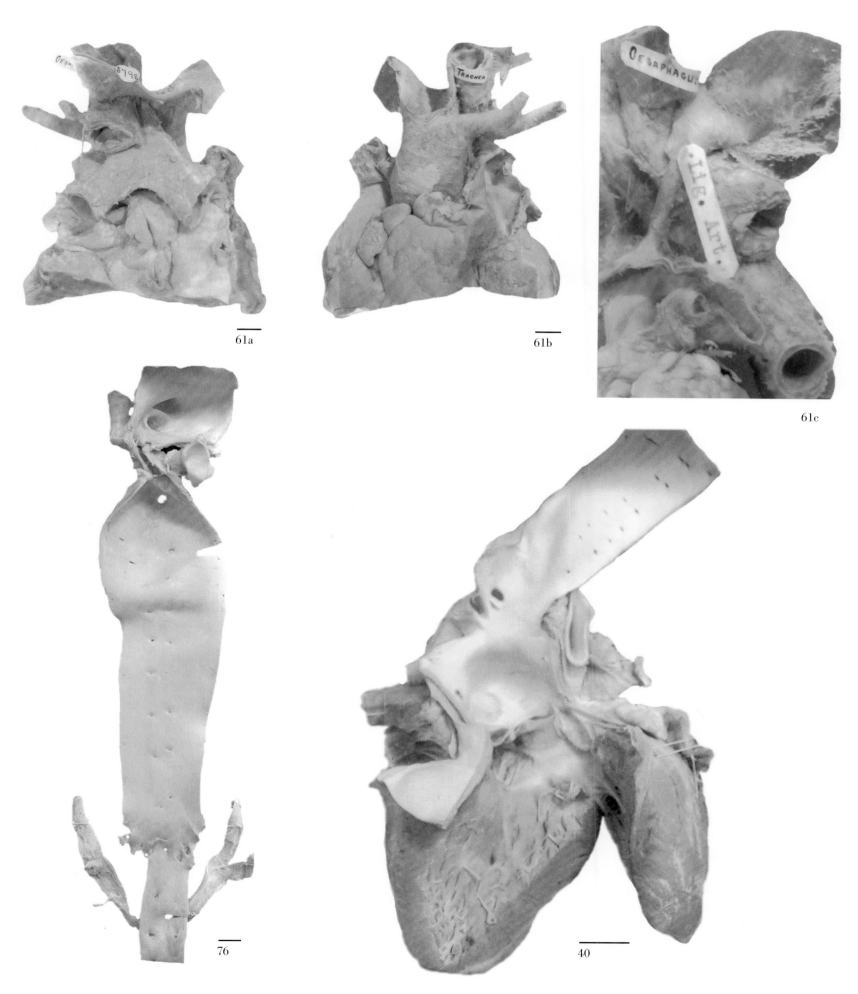

61a

61b

61c

76

40

61a, b, and c Right Aortic Arch. Ligamentum arteriosum passes backward from left to right for insertion in descending arch, forming a vascular ring encircling the trachea and esophagus (a − posterior; b − anterior; c − left lateral). *Atlas*, Plate VI Fig 6. 1914.

76 Coarctation of Aorta. Also mitral and tricuspid stenosis (not shown). Thirty-four-year-old woman, died 6 days post-partum. *Atlas*, Plate VIII, Fig 2. 1932.

40 Coarctation of Aorta. Patent foramen ovale (not shown); small ventricular septal defect. History unknown. 1907.

PLATE VII   ANOMALIES OF THE AORTIC VALVE

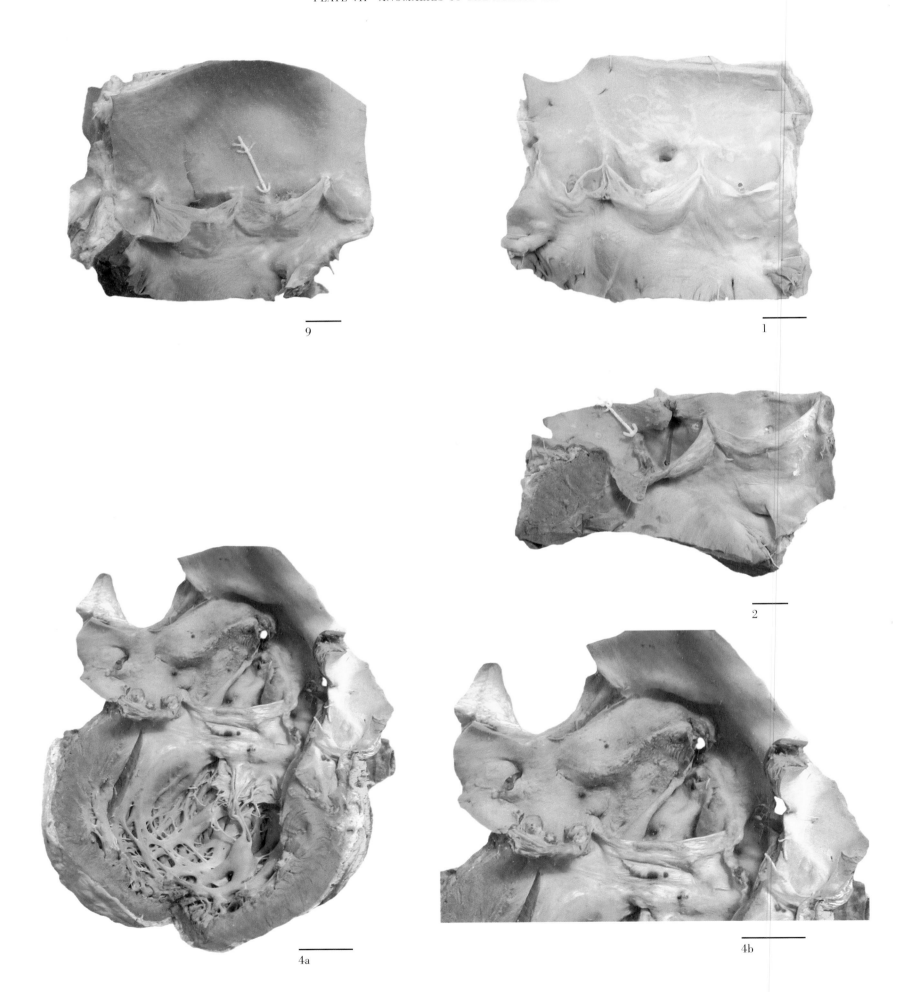

9

1

2

4a

4b

9 Supernumerary Aortic Segment,. Arrow points to raphe that partly separates aortic cusp. Fifty-year-old man. No cardiac symptoms. 1910.

1 Fenestrations of the Valve Cusp. Date unknown.

2 Fusion of Valve Cusps. 1906.

4a & b Bicuspid Aortic Valve. Ascending aorta tear with dissecting aneurysm. *Atlas*, Plate IX, Fig. 9. 1907.

PLATE VII   ANOMALIES OF THE AORTIC VALVE; ENDOCARDIAL ABNORMALITIES

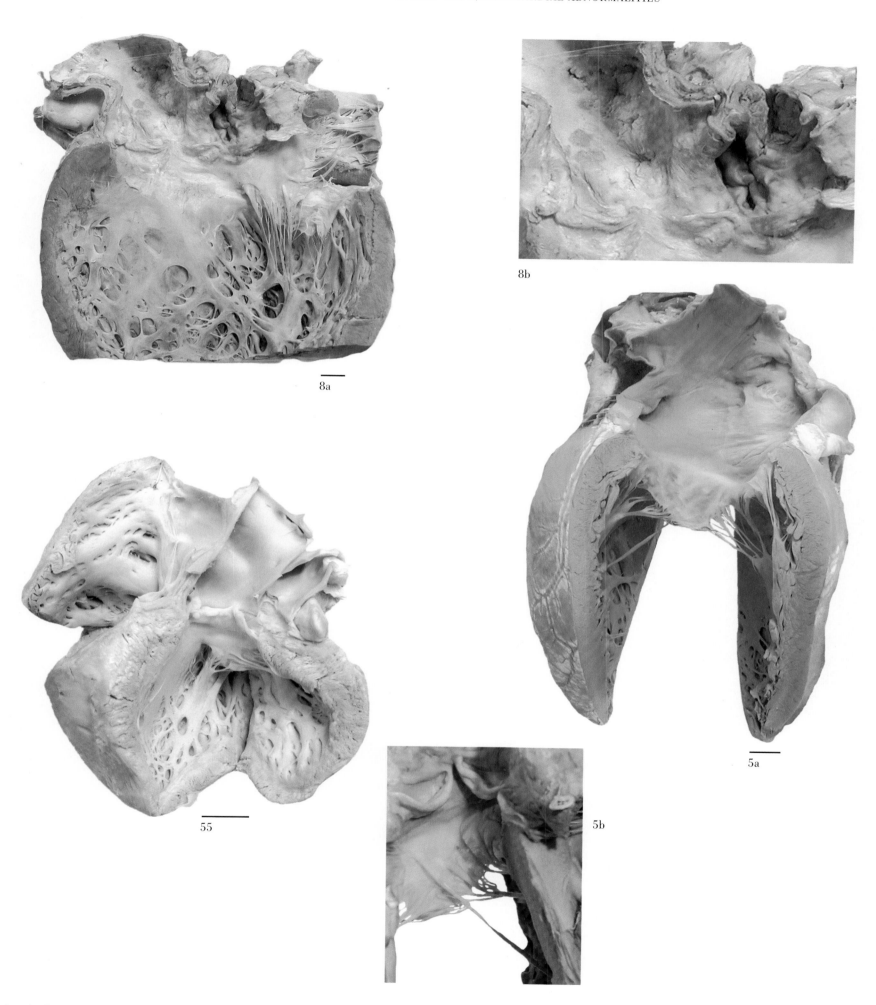

8a

8b

55

5a

5b

8a & b Super-numerary Aortic Cusp. Aneurysm of sinus of Valsalva (magnified in b). Syphilitic aortitis. Thirty-one-year-old man with aortic insufficiency. *Atlas*, Plate IX, Fig. 10. 1906.

55 Congenital Aortic Stenosis. Forty-seven-day-old infant. 1900.

5a & b Aberrant Chorda Tendiniae: a – left ventricle showing the anterior leaflet of mitral valve; b – magnified view of leaflet from behind showing band originating in the ventricular wall and inserting in the mid portion of the leaflet.

Fifty-year-old man with a mid-diastolic murmur attributed to the aberrant chorda. *Atlas*, Plate X, Fig. 2. 1899.

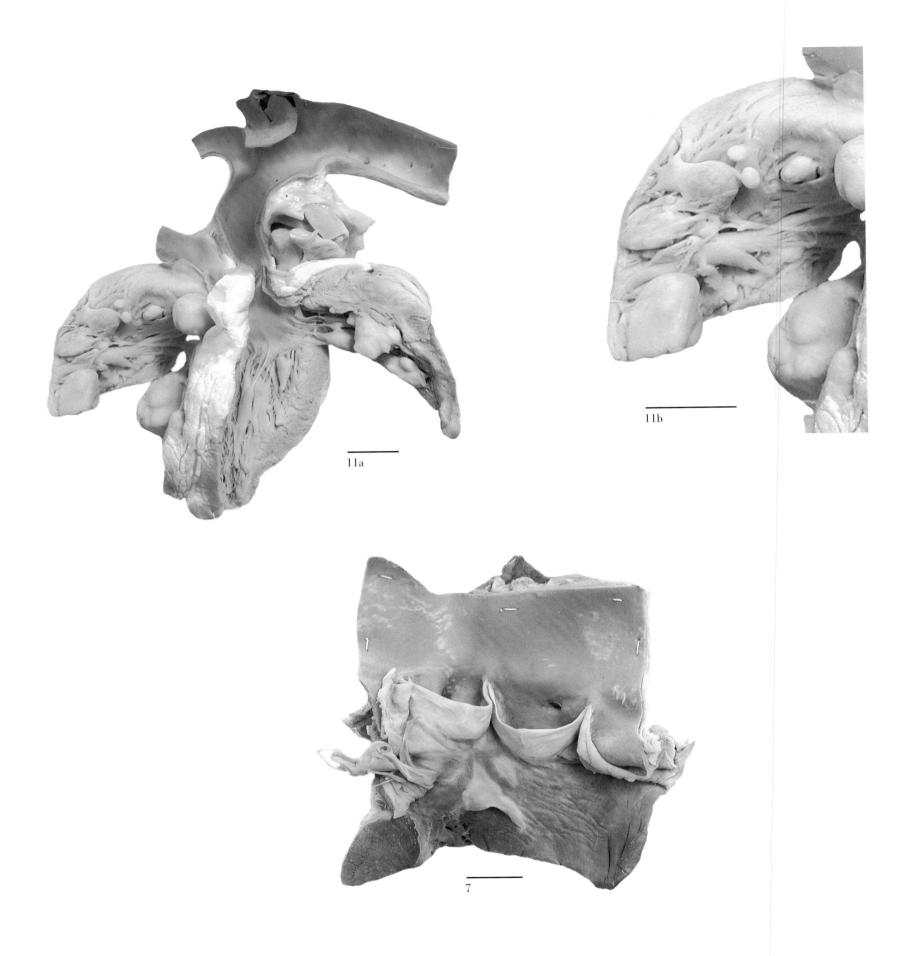

11a

11b

7

11a & b Congenital Rhabdomyoma.
Nine-month-old male infant with
tuberous sclerosis. *Atlas*, Plate XI,
Fig. 2. 1934.

7 Anomalous Endocardial Fold.
Anomalous fold situated below the angle
formed by the two coronary cusps,
resembling a reversed semilunar valve.
Incidental finding in a nineteen-year-old
man with miliary tuberculosis. 1910.

PLATE X   DUCTUS ARTERIOSUS: NORMAL FEATURES

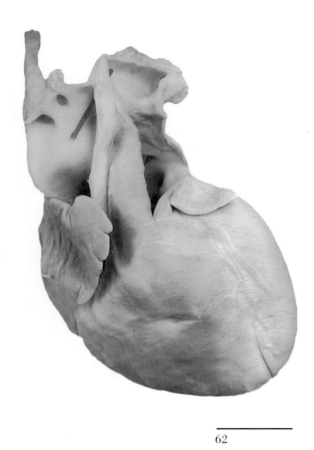

62

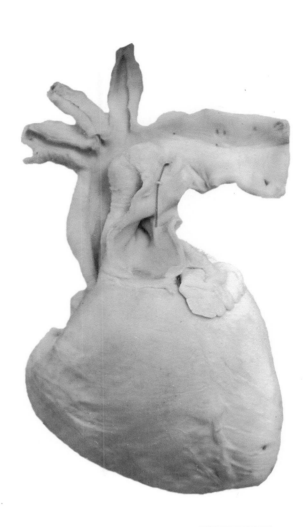

65

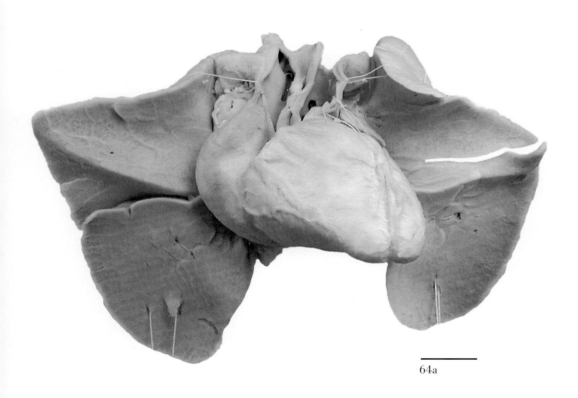

64a

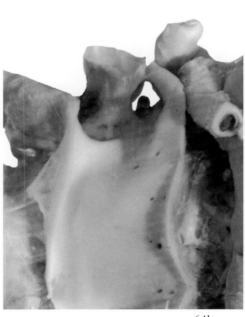

64b

62 Ductus Arteriosus. Premature infant born at eight months. 1909.

65 Ductus Arteriosus. Infant, three days after birth. 1909.

64a & b Ductus Arteriosus. Infant at birth: a – anterior view; b – posterior view. 1909.

PLATE XI   DUCTUS ARTERIOSUS: NORMAL FEATURES

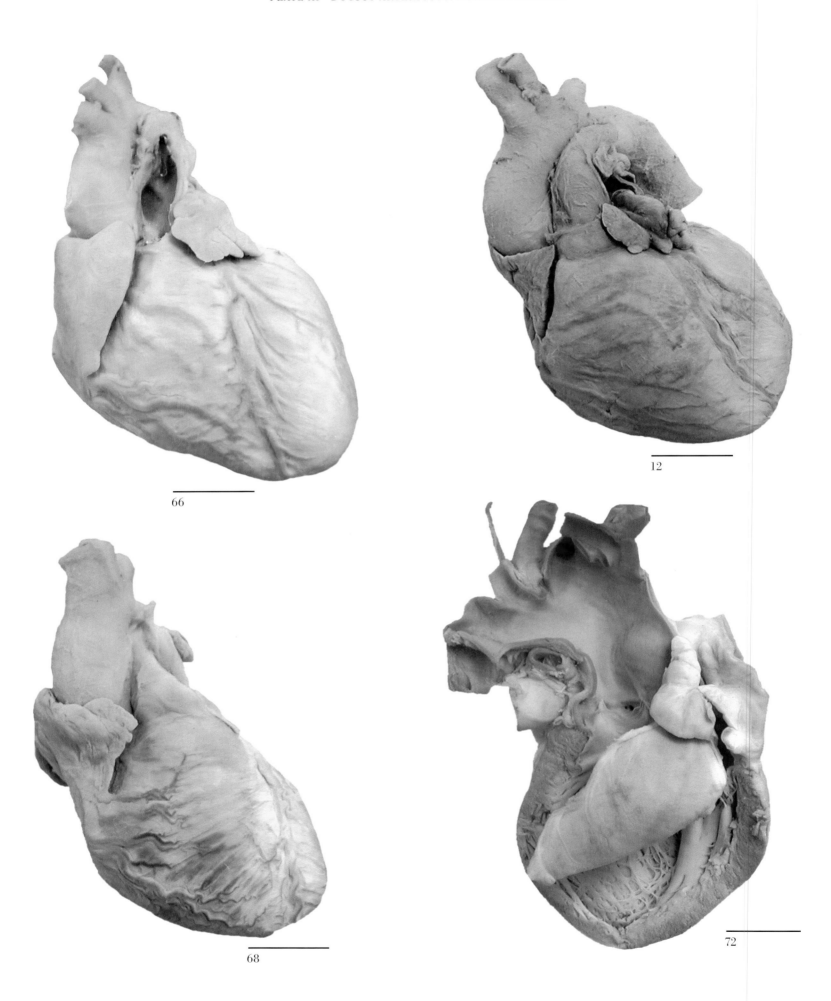

66 Ductus Arteriosus. Infant at six days. Ductus admits a probe. 1909.

12 Ductus Arteriosus. Infant at twenty days. Funnel-shaped aortic insertion. 1909.

68 Ductus Arteriosus. Infant at thirty-three days. Funnel-shaped aortic insertion. 1909.

72 Ductus Arteriosus. Infant at ten weeks. Ductus closed on aortic wall. Residual lumen evident as oval structure below isthmus. 1909.

PLATE XII   PATENT DUCTUS ARETRIOSUS

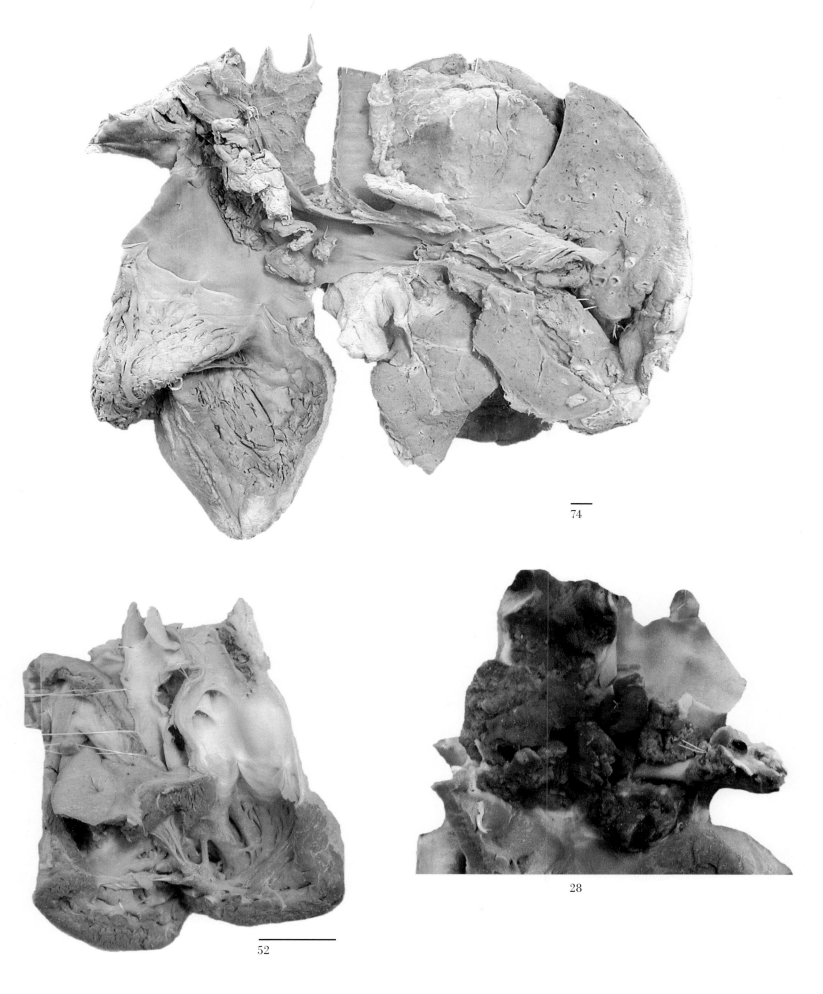

74

52

28

74 Patent Ductus Arteriosus with
Endocarditis. Nineteen-year-old woman
with ductal endocarditis and multiple
septic pulmonary emboli/abscesses
(Pneumococcus). *Atlas*, Plate XIII,
Fig. 4b. 1913.

52 Aortic Atresia. Widely patent ductus
connects hypoplastic aorta with dilated
pulmonary artery; marked right ventricular hypertrophy. Fifteen-day-old infant.
1913.

28 Pulmonary Artery and Ductus
Endocarditis. Large vegetations occlude
much of pulmonary trunk. Thirty-three-
year-old man, "symptomatic" for nine
months. 1921.

PLATE XIII   DEFECTS OF THE INTERAURICULAR SEPTUM

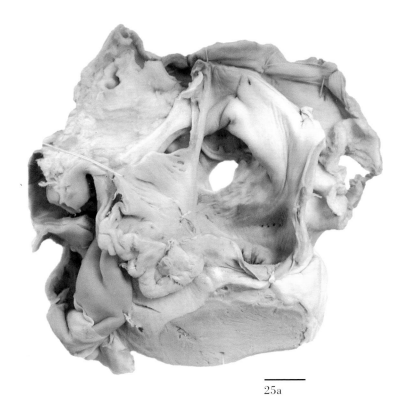

25a

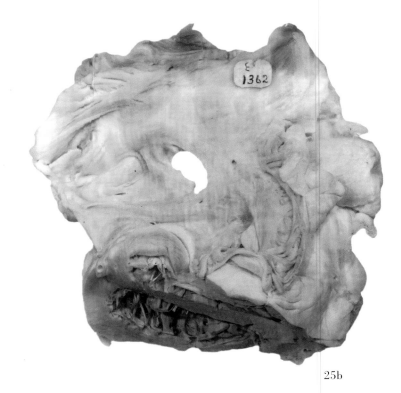

25b

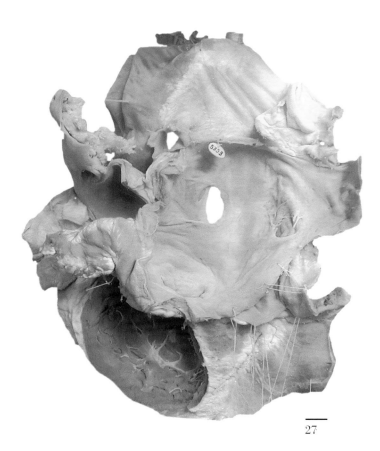

27

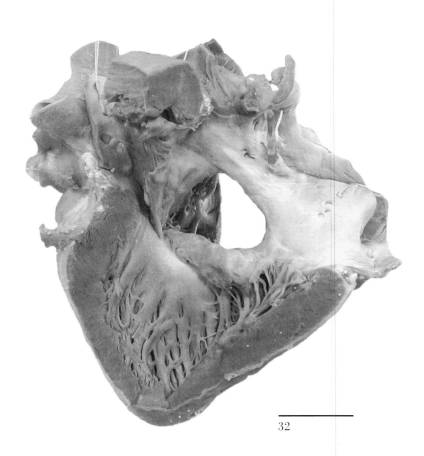

32

25a & b Patent Foramen Ovale. Biventricular hypertrophy and marked biatrial dilatation: a – right side; b – left side. Nineteen-year-old woman, history unknown. 1905.

27 Patent Foramen Ovale. Hemiplegia at age thirty. ? paradoxical embolism. Thirty-eight-year-old woman with history of "rheumatism" at age fourteen and multiple episodes of heart failure since twenty-eight. *Atlas*, Plate XIV, Fig 5. 1912.

32 Persistent Ostium Primum with Cleavage of Anterior Mitral Segment. Ten-month-old infant with Down Syndrome ("Mongolian idiot"). Death from bronchopneumonia. *Atlas*, Plate XIV, Fig. 8. 1922.

PLATE XIV   DEFECTS OF THE INTERAURICULAR SEPTUM

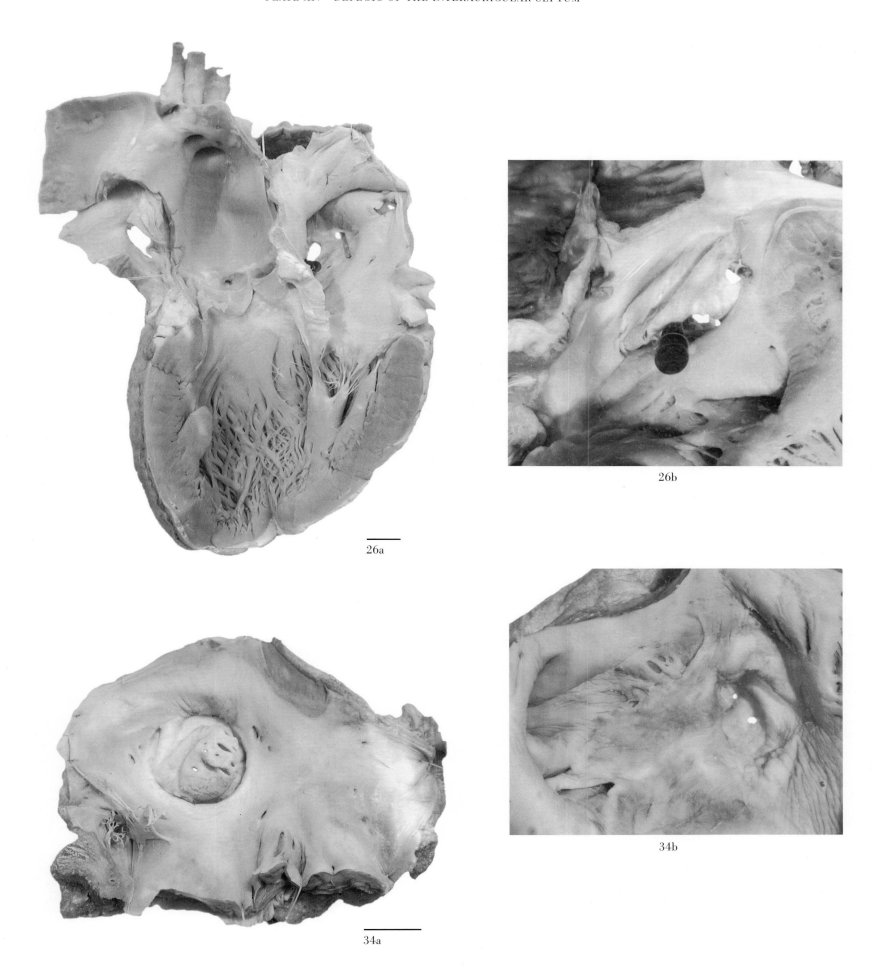

26a

26b

34a

34b

26a & b Patent Foramen Ovale: a – left ventricle and atrium; b – magnified view. Twenty-six-year-old woman, unknown history. 1914.

34a & b Cribriform Fossa Ovalis: a – right atrial side showing multiple fenestrations of membrane with bulging into chamber; b – appearance on left atrial side. Forty-seven-year-old man, unknown history. 1896.

PLATE XV   DEFECTS OF THE INTERVENTRICULAR SEPTUM

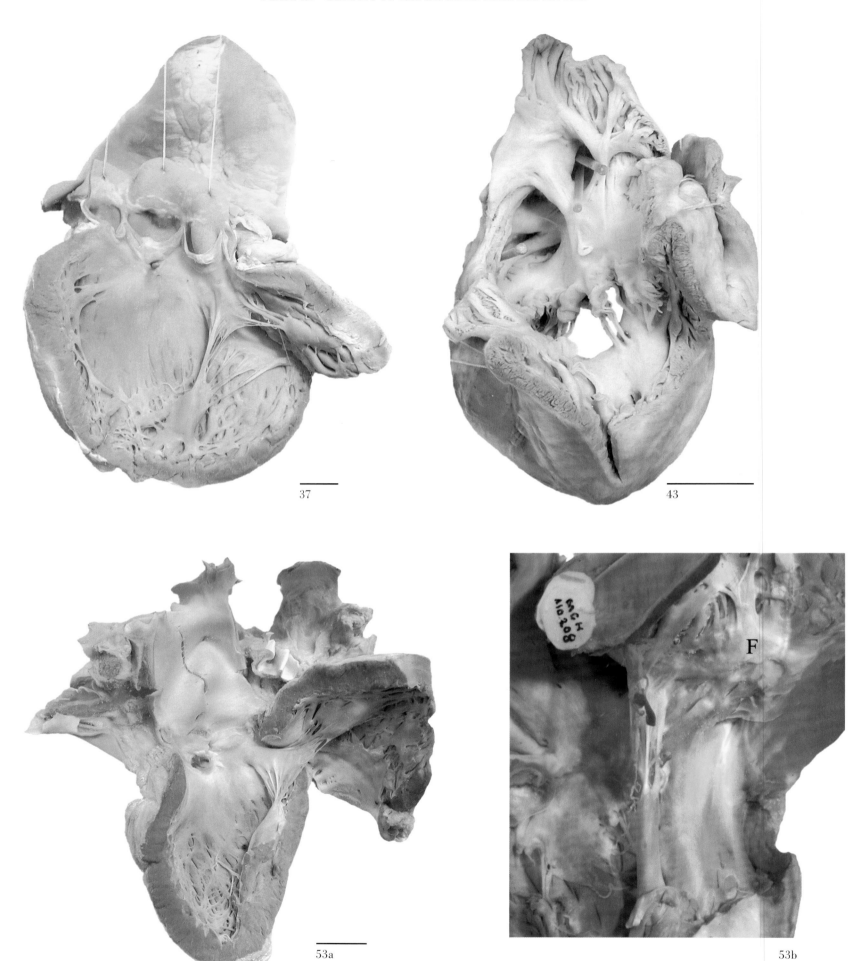

37

43

53a

F

53b

37 Small Defect of Interventricular Septum. Twenty-year-old woman, accidental death. *Atlas*, Plate XV, Fig. 3. Unknown date.

43 Defects of Interauricular and Interventricular Septa. Complete defect of interauricular septum (blue rods) and interventricular septum, with mitral and tricuspid valve anomalies ("incomplete double heart"). Ten-day-old girl. 1921.

53a & b Defect of Interventricular Septum with "Cicatrization": a – left side showing small defect (red rod) in the upper septum; b – right side, showing small focus of endocardial fibroelastosis; F opposite defect ("jet lesion"). Three-and-one-half-year-old boy, accidental death. 1910.

PLATE XVI   DEFECTS OF THE INTERVENTRICULAR SEPTUM

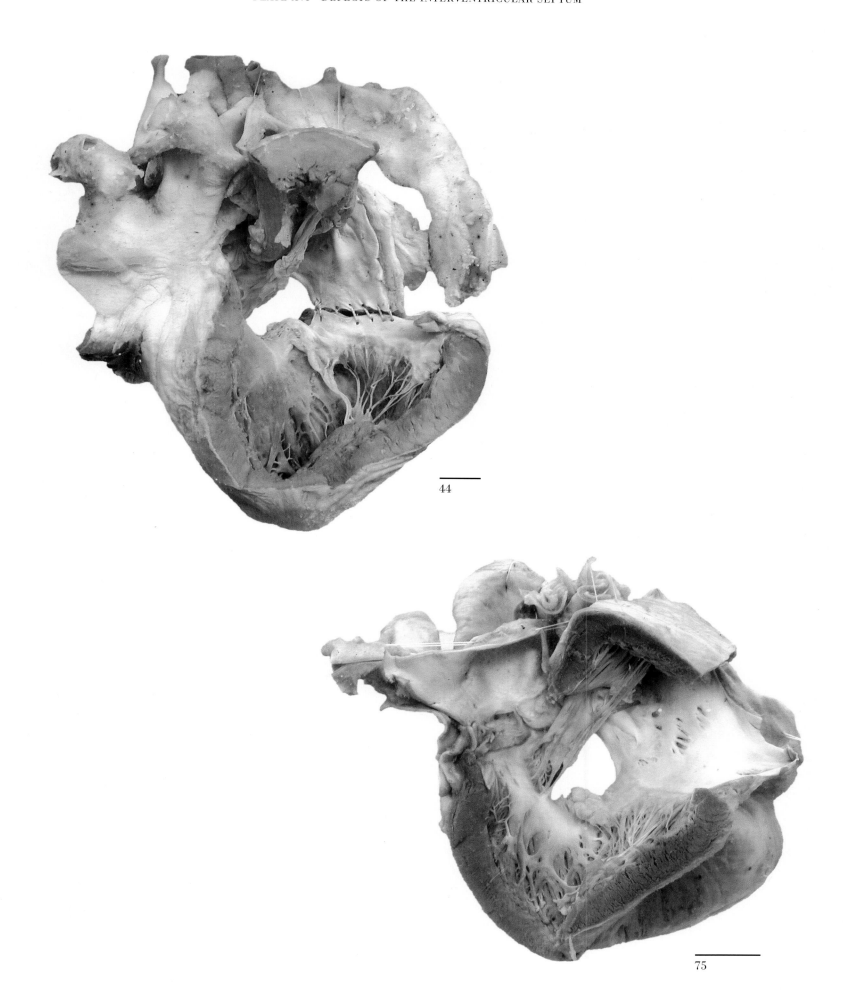

44

75

44 Persistent "Atrioventricular
Commune" with Cleavage of Mitral and
Tricuspid Segments. Transient cyanosis.
Four-and-one-half-year-old girl with
Down syndrome ("Mongolian idiot").
1931.

75 Common Atrioventricular Orifice
with Cleavage of Mitral and Tricuspid
Segments. Infant (unknown age) with
Down syndrome ("Mongolian idiot").
1914.

PLATE XVII   PULMONARY OUTFLOW TRACT STENOSIS

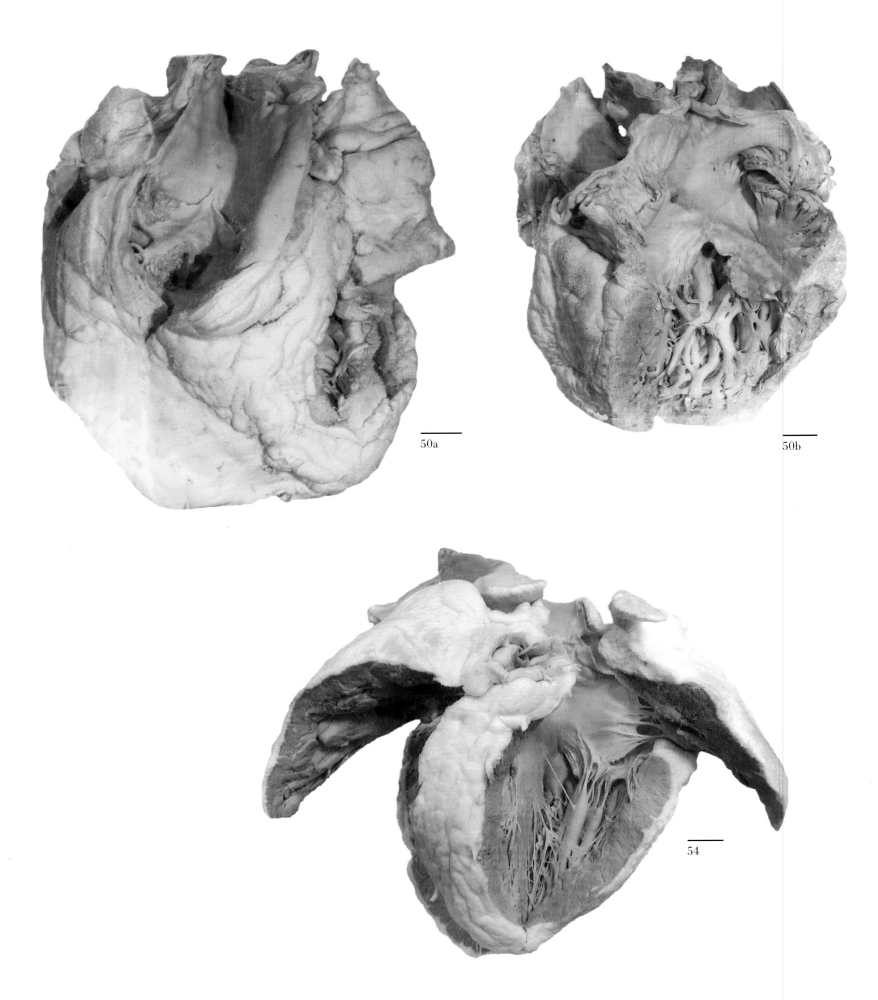

50a

50b

54

50a & b Stenosis of Right Ventricle at Lower Bulbar Orifice: a – separate conus chamber is open and shows finely granular endocarditis. Blue rod in outlet of right ventricle; b – right ventricular chamber with blue rod in orifice of conus chamber. Young woman with "signs of heart disease since childhood." *Atlas*, Plate XVII, Fig. 1. 1927

54 Pulmonary Valve Stenosis. Blue rod in funnel shaped pulmonary outflow tract. Large patent foramen ovale (not visible). Fourteen-year-old girl with dyspnea, cyanosis, and clubbing. *Atlas*, Plate XVIII, Fig. 5. 1921.

PLATE XVIII   PULMONARY STENOSIS/ATRESIA (TETRALOGY OF FALLOT)

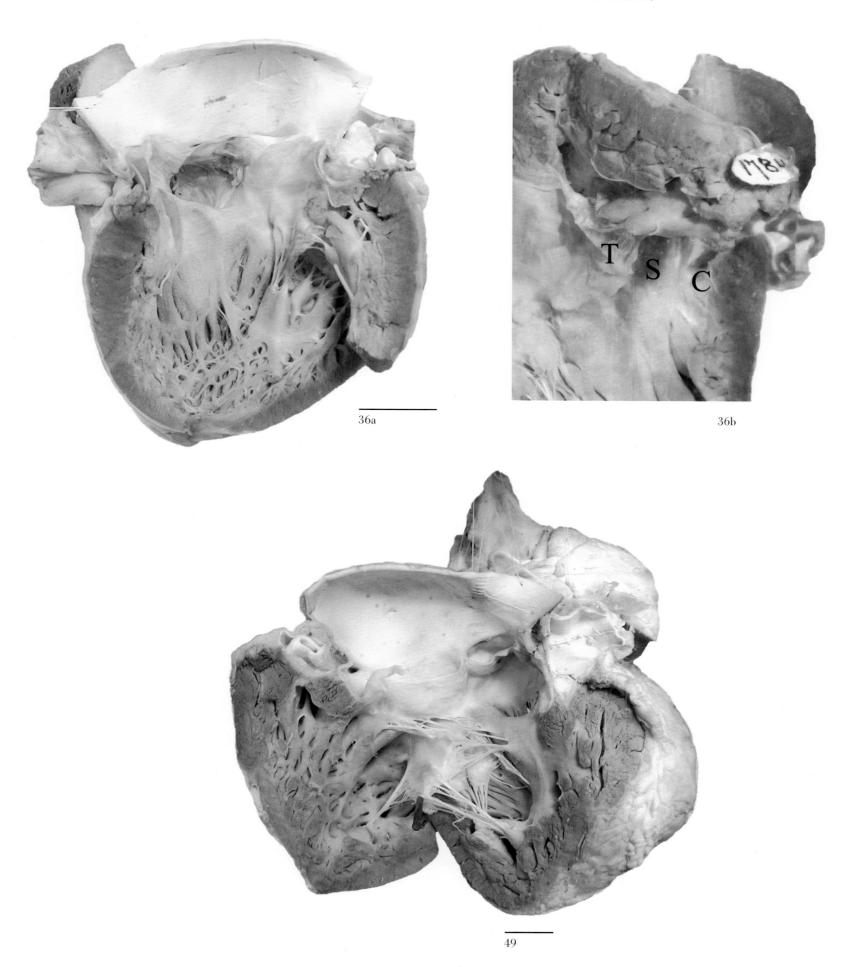

36a

36b

49

36a & b Tetralogy of Fallot: a – left ventricle showing dilated aorta and large interventricular septal defect; b – magnified view of right ventricle showing tricuspid valve leaflet; T septal defect; S and conus orifice; C infant, unknown age and date.

49 Tetralogy of Fallot. Left ventricle showing dilated aorta and orifice of interventricular septal defect. Stenotic pulmonary outflow tract is evident at left. Ten-year-old boy with cyanosis and hemiplegia. 1921.

PLATE XIX   PULMONARY STENOSIS/ATRESIA (TETRALOGY OF FALLOT)

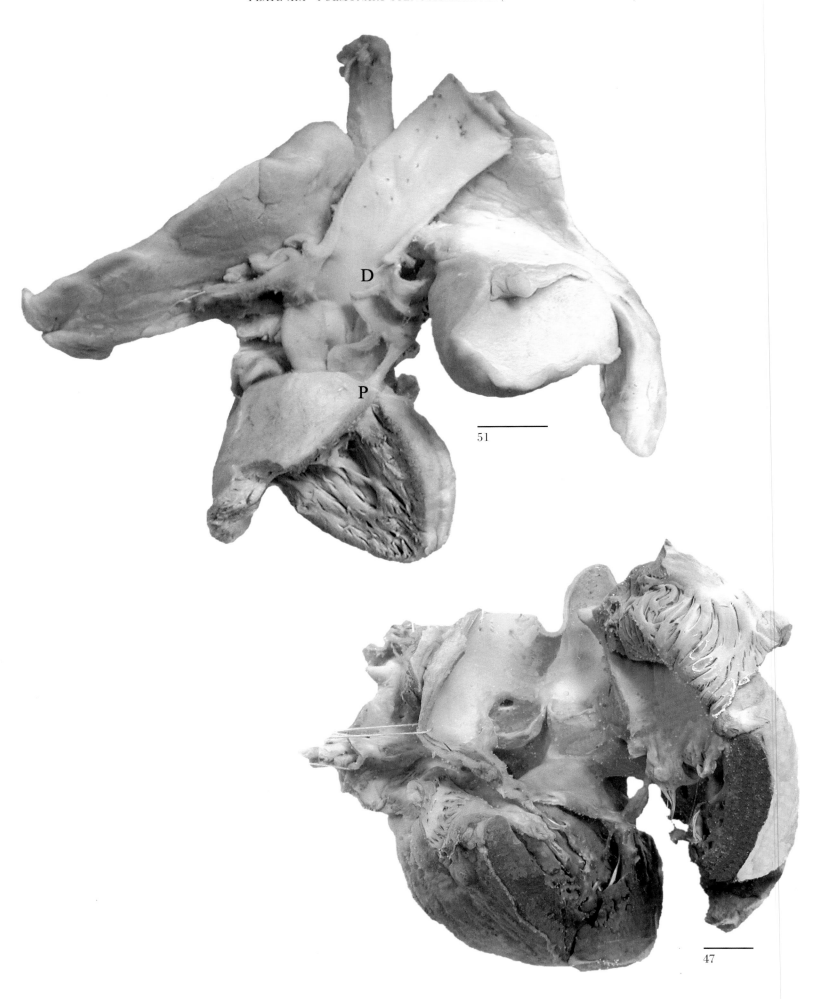

51 Tetralogy of Fallot. D patent ductus areteriosus; P origin of atretic pulmonary artery. Thirteen-day-old boy, cyanotic from birth. *Atlas*, Plate XIX, Fig. 6. c 1880.

47 Tetralogy of Fallot. Twelve-year-old girl with cyanosis and clubbing. 1903.

PLATE XX   COR TRILOCULARE: TRICUSPID ATRESIA

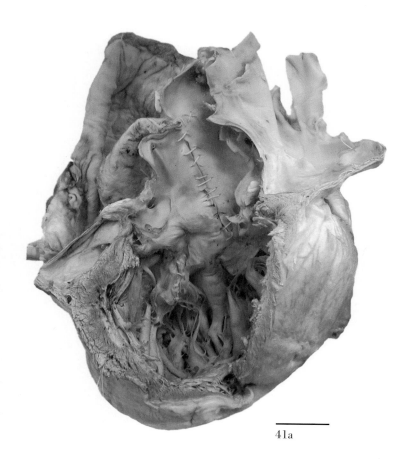

41a

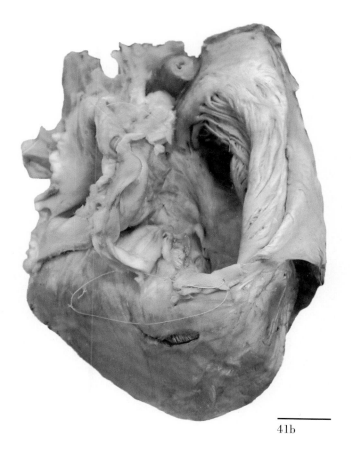

41b

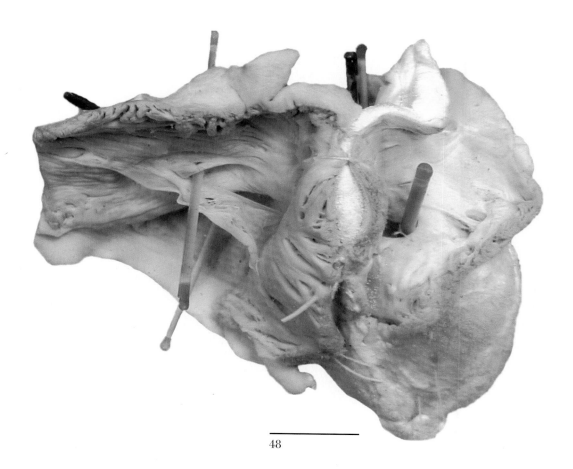

48

41a & b Cor Triloculare. Double-inlet left ventricle with persistent pulmonary conus (Holmes heart): a – left ventricular chamber and stitched aorta; b – left atrium. Twenty-two-year-old man with dyspnea and cyanosis. *Atlas*, Plate XXI, Fig. 6. 1823.

48 Tricuspid Atresia. View of right side of heart with patent foramen ovale (lower blue rod at left) and ventricular septal defect (blue rod at right projecting into right ventricle). Unknown age or history. 1923.

PLATE XXI   COMPLETE TRANSPOSITION OF GREAT TRUNKS

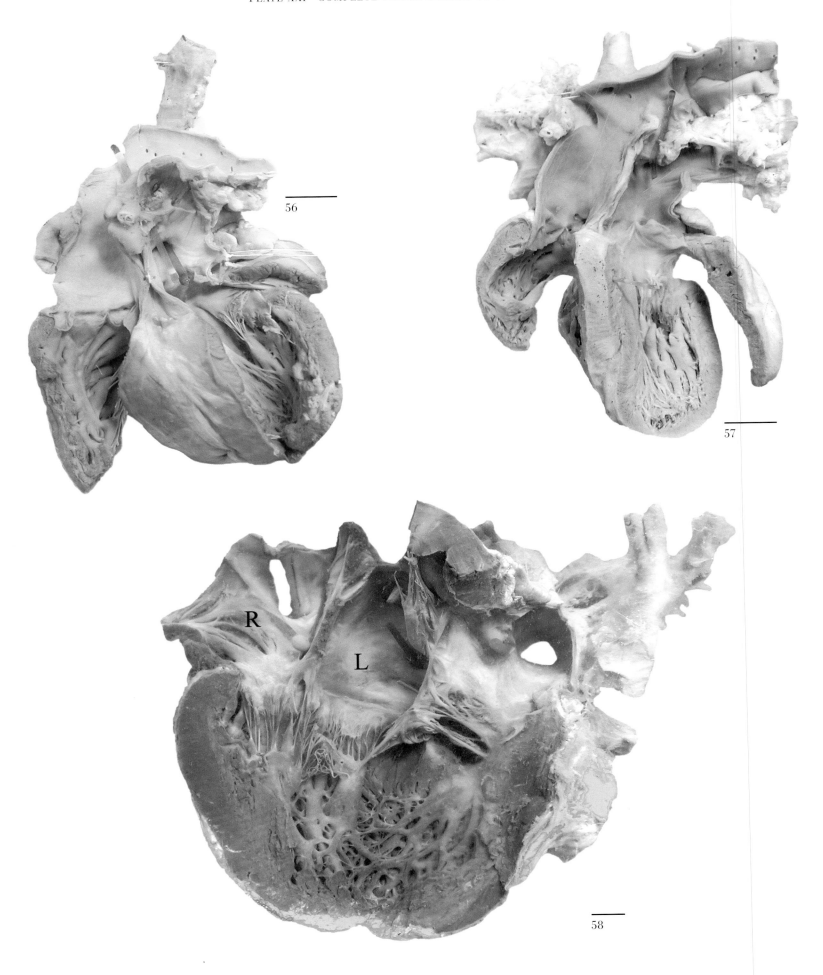

56 Complete Transposition of Arterial Trunks with Closed Ventricular Septum. Blue rod, patent ductus arteriosus; red rod, pulmonary artery. Patent foramen ovale not visible. Five-day-old infant with cyanosis and dyspnea. 1929.

57 Complete Transposition of Arterial Trunks with Small Ventricular Septal Defect. Red rod, patent ductus arteriosus; blue rod on right, ventricular septal defect. Patent foramen ovale not visible. Two-day-old infant, cyanotic from birth. 1934.

58 Complete Transposition of Arterial Trunks with Ventricular Septal Defect. Patent ductus arteriosus and stenosis of conus of right ventricle (not visible). Double mitral orifice; R right atrium; L left atrium. Twenty-year-old man with cyanosis and dyspnea from childhood.

Died of massive pulmonary hemorrhage. *Atlas*, Plate XXIV, Fig. 3. 1929.

PLATE XXII   MISCELLANEOUS ANOMALIES

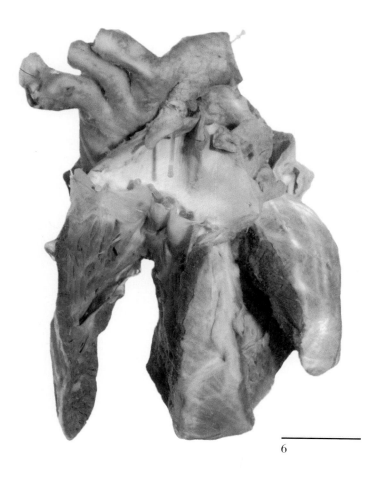

6

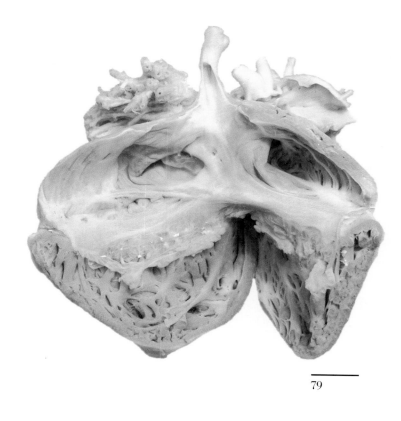

79

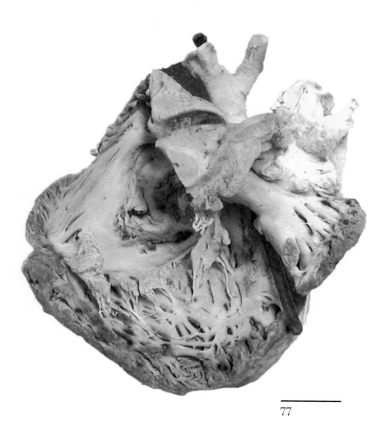

77

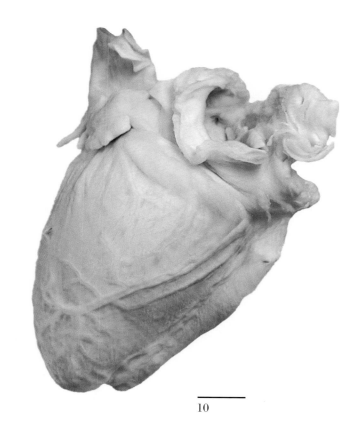

10

6 Surpernumerary Pulmonary Valve Cusp. Blue rod in patent ductus arteriosus. Fourteen-week-old infant. 1908.

79 Absence of Papillary Muscles Tricuspid Valve. Neonatal death (one hour). 1935.

77 Absence of aortic Arch. Red rod through aortic valve directly into great vessels to the neck. Unknown age; Down syndrome ("Mongolian idiot"). 1929.

10 Bifid Apex. The apex of each ventricle projects downward about 5 mm below the interventricular groove. Eight-year-old child, died of diabetes. 1899.

ATLAS OF
CONGENITAL CARDIAC DISEASE

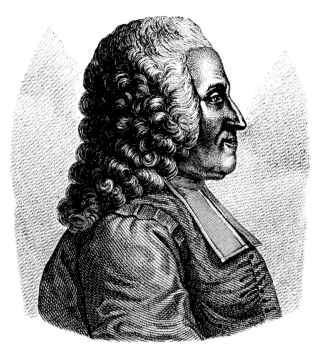

Jean-Baptiste de Sénac
(1693–1770)

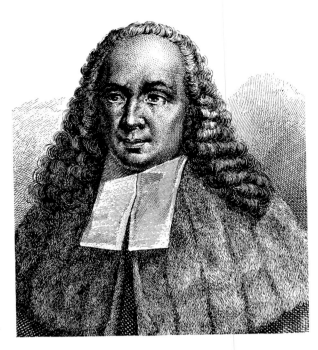

Giovanni Baptista Morgagni
(1682–1771)

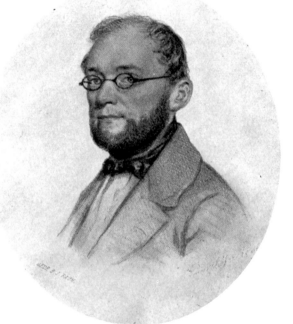

Carl Rokitansky
(1804–1878)

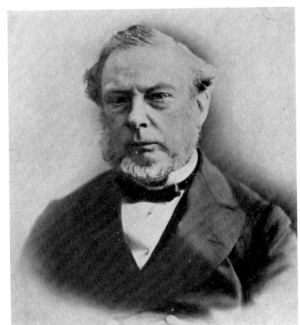

Thomas B. Peacock (1812–1882)

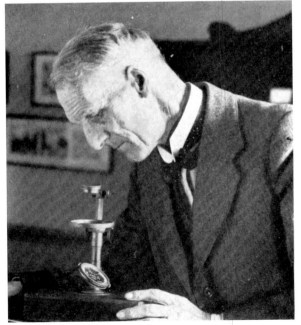

Sir Arthur Keith (1866–   )

(Frontispiece.)

Great Scientists Who Have Made Fundamental Contributions to Our
Knowledge of Congenital Heart Disease

ATLAS

OF

CONGENITAL CARDIAC DISEASE

BY

MAUDE E. ABBOTT, B.A., M.D., F.R.C.P. (Canada)

Curator of the Historical Medical Museum and
Assistant Professor of Medical Research
McGill University,
Montreal, Canada

Published by

THE AMERICAN HEART ASSOCIATION

50 WEST 50TH STREET, NEW YORK, N.Y.

1936

PRINTED IN CANADA

FOREWORD

Sénac, Peacock, Rokitansky, and Keith, one after the other, richly advanced our knowledge of congenital heart disease, but it was left to Maude Abbott, fired by a spark from Osler, to make the subject one of such general and widespread interest that we no longer regard it with either disdain or awe as a mystery for the autopsy table alone to discover and to solve. She has been the most important of the pioneers in establishing congenital heart disease as a living part of clinical medicine.

For a long time the medical world has awaited a textbook on congenital heart disease by Dr. Abbott, whose contributions in this field have up to this time been accessible only in her system-monographs or in the periodical literature. In assembling her material in preparation for a future work of such importance she presented a notable exhibit before the Centennial Meeting of the British Medical Association in London in 1934 and again before the Joint Meeting of the American and Canadian Medical Associations in Atlantic City in 1935 and before the Ontario Medical Association in 1936. It is this exhibit with some modifications and additions that has been put into permanent and convenient form as an Atlas.

PAUL D. WHITE.

BOSTON, MASS.
July, 1936.

INTRODUCTION

This volume presents, in a somewhat unusual form, a pictorial retrospect of the author's personal experience in what may now be considered a specialized field of clinico-pathological research. A first-hand knowledge of the exact morphology of a large range of cardiac anomalies, obtained in the first place through an intensive early study of the rich material accumulated under the author's care as Curator of the Medical Museum of McGill University, has been continuously applied and amplified through more than three decades of activity, by observation of congenital heart disease in the wards and autopsy rooms of many great hospitals both at home and abroad. Of recent years, also, an ever-increasing consultant correspondence has grown up between the writer and clinicians in many parts of this continent, who have sent in their material, often unique of its kind, to the McGill Museum for description and diagnosis. This circumstance has brought a wider range of these rare conditions under personal notice than would have been otherwise possible and has thus supplied a large opportunity for the evaluation of the various aspects of this subject and the segregation in it of the different clinical types into which these conditions naturally fall. The flood of recent literature and the more exact data now available through modern laboratory methods have been likewise conducive to the clearer understanding of this subject, which is only now coming into its own as a field of vital human interest. It is, however, a well-recognized fact that, in clinical medicine, the intimate personal knowledge of a relatively small number of individual cases is likely to yield a richer harvest in the understanding of diseased conditions than wider generalizations covering a more vast material. The concentration upon the clinical picture presented by his own carefully studied patients was the source of Sydenham's contribution to the nosology of disease; and Osler himself looked back upon the 750 autopsies performed by himself at the Montreal General Hospital as the very foundation stones of his career. In the intriguing subject before us, the study of each individual case is indeed the sole key to the comprehension of these obscure conditions, in the investigation of which "the music of the spheres" is dimly perceptible behind the inevitable fulfillment of ontogenetic and teleologic laws. It is, therefore, this service which the present Atlas seeks to render to the student, in placing before him, in objective form, the actual morphological substratum of the experience of a single individual worker. Not all the cases presented were the author's "own," in the narrower sense of the term, but all, even those culled from the writings of the great observers of an earlier generation, may be considered, through the writer's intimate familiarity with their detail and con-

tent, a personal observation, in the deeper meaning of the term. The conditions illustrated here represent a fairly complete range of those cardiac anomalies "of clinical significance" observed to date, the only serious omissions (made for lack of space) being those of congenital pulmonary dilatation (on which see B. S. Oppenheimer, *Tr. Assn. Amer. Phys.*, 1933, **48**: 290) and pericardial defect (reviewed by the writer in Osler's *Modern Medicine*, 1927, **4**: 657).

A short autobiographical statement, relating how the writer's attention was first drawn to this extraordinarily interesting subject, the part which Sir William Osler took in rendering effective her early work in this field, and the evolution of the research itself will be, we believe, in place here. Appointed to the curatorship of the McGill Museum in the year 1899, just after her return from two years' preliminary training in Internal Medicine and Pathology under Ortner and Kolisko in Vienna, the author became at once interested in an unlabeled specimen in the collection. This was a three-chambered adult heart presenting an anomalous septum cutting off a small supplementary cavity, from which arose the (untransposed) pulmonary artery (Pl. XXI, Fig. 6a). At the suggestion of the late Professor Wyatt Johnston (himself a museum enthusiast), an inquiry was addressed to Dr. Osler, then in Baltimore, asking whether he could identify the case. He replied promptly that he remembered the specimen perfectly, having often demonstrated it to students during his professoriate at McGill, and that it had been reported in an early Edinburgh journal by "old Dr. Andrew Holmes" (first Dean of the McGill Medical Faculty). The writer accordingly located the article in the *Transactions of the Edinburgh Medico-Chirurgical Society* in 1824, where it appeared with a fine copper plate engraving of the heart, and learned from it that the autopsy on this case (which is still unique in the literature of cardiac anomalies) was performed by Dr. Holmes at the Montreal General Hospital in 1823, the year of the foundation of the McGill Medical School, in the presence of the other three founders of that institution. This remarkable combination of interesting features and circumstances led to her republication, in 1901, of Dr. Holmes's report along with his engraving of the heart and a semidiagrammatic sketch of the circulation by Dr. R. Tait Mackenzie (Pl. XXI, Fig. 6b), together with a biographical sketch of this early clinico-pathologist, who is one of the most important and interesting figures in the medical history of that period on this continent. It was this semihistorical, semipathological article, together with the writer's activities in the cataloguing of the Pathological Collection made by Dr. Osler during his term as Pathologist to the Montreal General Hospital and housed at that time under her care in the Museum, that led Sir William, in 1905, to extend to her the invitation to write a section on Congenital Cardiac Disease in his new *System of Modern Medicine*. He himself suggested that the subject might be treated "statistically" and the first edition of this monograph accordingly contained a chart of 412 cases of congenital heart disease with autopsies analyzed from the literature. Fully one-third of these were drawn from the *Transactions of the Pathological Society of London*, that goldmine of early clinico-pathological observation, and Vierordt's great monograph, which had appeared shortly before this and was actually the first which had handled the subject from the statistical standpoint, was used as a guide and sourcebook throughout.

Dr. Osler received the proof of the first edition of this monograph at his home in Oxford in January, 1908. With his characteristic generosity toward younger workers, and with the insight that impelled him to the instant recognition of what he believed to be a contribution of scientific merit, he immediately sent off a letter to the writer expressing his warm approval of its contents.

In the second edition of Osler and McCrae's *System*, which appeared in 1915, the number of cases analyzed by the writer was raised to 631, and in its third edition published in 1927, there were 850 cases analyzed. In 1924 another monograph by the writer on the Treatment of Congenital Heart Disease appeared, and in 1928, one on the diagnosis of this condition (Part 1 with Dr. E. Weiss), and finally in 1932, in *Nelson's Loose-leaf Medicine*, a fourth, containing a review of the recent literature on this subject from the publication of the third edition of Osler and McCrae's *System* in 1927 to that date, with a chart of 1,000 cases analyzed (republished here by kind permission of Thomas Nelson & Sons). Finally, the Atlas here published is merely preliminary to a larger volume on congenital heart disease which the author has under preparation. In its objective presentation of the individual cases studied, it has, we believe, a supplementary function of real value, which only a publication of this type can adequately fulfill.

The writer's sincerest thanks are expressed to the American Heart Association for their valuable support in their publication of this Atlas and especially to Dr. H. M. Marvin, Executive Chairman, and Miss Gertrude Wood, Office Secretary, for their courtesy and cooperation; to Dr. Paul White and his staff and the many other contributors who have placed their unpublished cases so freely at the writer's disposal for publication here; to Mr. Lucius N. Littauer of the Littauer Foundation for financial support kindly given for the preparation for publication of the writer's researches in this field; and to Dr. Maurice Kugel for his generous action in the same regard; to Messrs. Lea and Febiger and the other publishers and the medical artists mentioned in the text, whose original drawings and fine reproductions embellish these pages; to Dr. David Seecof of the Jewish Hospital of Montreal for kind assistance in the photographic and other preliminary work incidental to the inception of this Atlas and to Dr. Otto Kruger for his valuable help in the construction of the plates; and, last but not least, to the writer's efficient secretary, Miss Edna F. Graham, with whose help and faithful cooperation this Atlas and the exhibits upon which it is based have attained their present adequate form.

Maude E. Abbott.

Montreal, Canada.
July 15, 1936.

TABLE OF CONTENTS

PART I
DEVELOPMENT AND COMPARATIVE ANATOMY OF THE HEART

PLATE I

DEVELOPMENT OF THE REPTILIAN AND MAMMALIAN HEART

An understanding of the elementary facts of human and comparative embryology is essential to an intelligent grasp of the ontogenetic problems of congenital cardiac disease. In the light of a knowledge of the successive stages through which the mammalian heart passes in its evolution from its primitive tubular state to the completely divided four-chambered organ conducting a double circulation, the most bizarre combinations of defects can usually be interpreted quite simply, as due to early arrests of development, marked it may be by ingenious structural adaptations of growth. The critical period in the human subject lies between the fifth and eighth weeks of embryonic life, i.e., before the cardiac septa are formed, and while the complex processes of torsion, involution, readjustment and fusion are taking place at the base, interruption of which is the source of most of the graver anomalies. The figures shown opposite have been selected with a view to illustrating this particular stage in development, which is of particular interest in view of the modern phylogenetic theories on the ontogenesis of the graver cardiac defects.

For a complete survey of this subject see the accounts by T. Walmsley, *Quain's Anatomy*, 1929, IV, Pt. III: 3–20; 37–41; 59–62; 97–108; *Cunningham's Anatomy*, 6th ed., 1931, 26–34; 1040–1046; also Keith, *Human Embryology and Morphology*, 1921; Tandler's article in Keibel and Mall, *Embryology*, 1912, II; 534–570; and that by D. Waterston on "The development of the heart in man," *Tr. Roy. Soc. Edin.*, 1912, **52**: 257.

Fig. 1.—Microphotograph of a transverse section through the heart of a 10-mm. pig embryo. Note the sinus venosus above on the right, emptying into the right auricle between the valvulae venosae dextra et sinistra; the large auricles pouching forward on either side above and completely divided by the septum primum which has united below with the auricular ventricular cushions (septum intermedium) and is perforated above by the foramen ovale. The septum secundum has not yet developed. The large ventricular part with a spongy musculature and bifid apex lies below. The interventricular septum is incomplete, leaving a large defect at its upper border between the right and left chambers; the mitral and tricuspid ostia are still lined by embryonic endocardial cushions (rudimentary valves). (From a serial section made by Alton Maturin of the Harvard Medical School.)

Fig. 2.—Reconstruction models of the interior of the hearts of two turtle embryos at different stages of development, showing the gradual division of the conus into three separate vessels, the reptilian right and left aortae and the pulmonary artery.

a. From a 9-mm. turtle embryo (earlier stage). The third and fourth pairs of aortic arches emerge at the top of the model, and just below these are the conal ridges, which have not yet met and are seen as deep grooves leaving high crests between each which will later form the lumina of the three separate vessels seen in Fig. 2b below. In the bulbar region the right ridge predominates and twists spirally to assume a left central position. (From the models by J. L. Bremer, Pl. 5, Fig. 12; Pl. 6, Fig. 11. Reference under Fig. 4d.)

b. From a turtle embryo of 16.8 mm. Here division has been completed by union of the conal ridges (Fig. 2a above) and the three vessels are seen emerging separately from the bulbar region below.

Fig. 3.—Early stages in the development of the heart of Lacerta agilis.

1. Heart tube from embryo of 0.4 mm., showing curve to right between the fixed cranial (arterial) end above and the caudal (venous) end below.

2 and 3. Heart tube from embryo of 0.6 mm., ventral and lateral aspects. The tube is now S shaped from the turning up of the venous end. *I.l.A.B.*, first left aortic arch.

4 and 5. The same. From an embryo of 0.9 mm. Venous end rising posteriorly on the left. In the lateral view the sinus venosus (+-+) is seen receiving the duct of Cuvier (*D.C.s*) above and the omphalo-mesenteric vein (*V.o.m.s.*) below.

6 and 7. The same. From an embryo of 1.2 mm. The auricle (*At.*) is seen in the lateral view (7) to be rising above the ventricular part of the heart.

8. Heart and truncus arteriosus (*T.art.*) from embryo of 2 mm. The auricle has now risen above the ventricle to the left of the bulbus cordis. Note the deep bulbo-auricular (*S.b.aur.*) and bulbo-ventricular (*Kn.F.*) clefts.

9. The same, with a slice removed at the line marked *XY* in 8, showing the interior. Note distal (*d.B.W.* II and IV) and proximal (*p.B.W.A.* and *B.*) bulbar swellings at level of aortic cusps and conus orifice, radial trabecular system (*r.T.S.*), endocardial cushions (*E.K.*) at auriculo-ventricular orifice, and torsion of bulbar cavity. (From Greil, "Anatomy and development of the heart and truncus arteriosus in reptiles," *Morphol. Jahrb.*, 1903, **31**: 128–130; 304, Pl. VI.)

Fig. 4.—Reconstruction models or casts of interior of the embryonic heart showing the progressive torsion that takes place clockwise or dextral at its arterial and sinistral at its venous end, and the gradual differentiation of chambers, development of septa and division of great trunks.

a. Model of cavities of heart of chick embryo of 50 hours incubation. Flattened S-shaped tube curving to right with venous end entering on the left posteriorly and the aortic arches arising from the bulbar enlargement at right upper angle.

b. The same at 4 days 12 hours. The auricles have risen and pouch forward. Septum primum appears as a cleft above posteriorly on the left leaving a large ostium primum (seen as a solid mass) below. The auriculo-ventricular cushions (seen as cavity) separate the mitral and tricuspid orifices (seen as wax lines). The bulbar end has undergone a marked clockwise torsion toward the median line before giving off the aortic arches above. The ventricle has been cut away below and is represented by projections indicating clefts between the trabeculae.

c. The same at 5 days incubation. The auricles are greatly enlarged with corrugated surfaces (indicating clefts) and divided below by the septum primum which has met the auriculo-ventricular cushions (seen as cavity). The still undivided bulbus lies obliquely in the median line anteriorly and gives off the aorta and pulmonary artery.

d. The same at 5 days 15 hours. The upper part of the auricles and the lower part of the ventricles have been cut away. Complete division of the auricles, ventricles and great trunks has now occurred. Patent foramen ovale in auricular septum. Note that through the spiral torsion that takes place in the bulbus (Fig. 2a) the pulmonary rises on the extreme left anteriorly and the aorta on the right posteriorly. These are the normal postnatal relations. (Republished by permission from J. L. Bremer, "Interpretation of development of the heart. The left aorta of reptiles," *Amer. J. Anat.*, 1928, **42**: 307, Pl. 2, Fig. 3; Pl. 3, Fig. 6; Pl. 4, Fig. 8; Pl. 5, Fig. 9.)

PLATE I. DEVELOPMENT OF THE REPTILIAN AND MAMMALIAN HEART

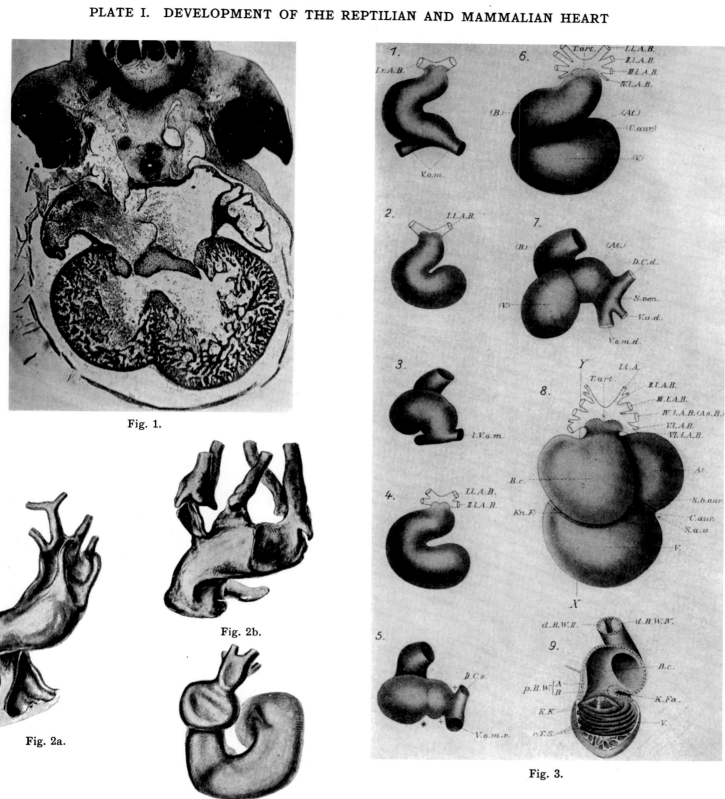

Fig. 1.

Fig. 2a.

Fig. 2b.

Fig. 4a.

Fig. 3.

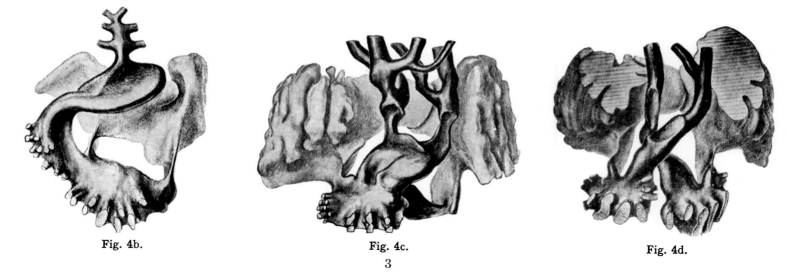

Fig. 4b.

Fig. 4c.

Fig. 4d.

PLATE II

COMPARATIVE ANATOMY. FISH AND AMPHIBIAN HEART

Much light is cast upon the development of the mammalian heart, and, incidentally, upon the period at which arrest of growth has taken place in cardiac anomalies of the graver sort by a comparative study of the adult fish, amphibian and reptilian organ. The truly extraordinary way in which these various orders in the ascending vertebrate scale mirror the successive stages through which the human heart passes in very early intrauterine life is one of nature's most spectacular and impressive feats, presenting as it does a complete review of this organ's evolution down to the closure of the cardiac septa in the eighth week of foetal life. The correlation of cases of cardiac defect with these fields of embryology and comparative anatomy becomes especially instructive in view of the fact that steps evanescent in the human embryo, but fixed in its phylogenetic prototype, are not infrequently revealed in the anomaly, caught in flight as it were at the moment of the arrest. The earlier stages of development of the human embryo where the heart is an undivided tubular organ with ventricular bend to the right (Pl. I) are thus mirrored in the primitive heart of the teleost fish, in which there are four chambers arranged caudo-cranially, namely, sinus venosus, common auricle, common ventricle and bulbus cordis (Fig. 1). There is no sign of subdivision into right and left halves, except possibly at the extreme caudal extremity, which has risen posteriorly in the higher fish orders and pouches forward above the ventricle (Figs. 2–3). Similar conditions prevail in the amphibian heart, except that here subdivision into lateral chambers is actually beginning caudally, both in the roof of the auricle and at the entrance of the sinus venosus (Fig. 5).

The illustrations opposite of fish and amphibian hearts (Figs. 1, 2, and 5) and also those of the python heart (Pl. III, Figs. 4a and b) are from drawings of specimens in the Cardiac Anomaly Collection of the Medical Museum of McGill University, made by the late W. W. Beattie and E. Shanly and published with the writer in "Cardiac defects in the light of comparative anatomy," *J. Tech. Meth.*, 1922, **8**: 188. Figure 3 is from Jane Robertson's brilliant contribution on the development of spiral torsion in the bulbus cordis of the higher orders of fish hearts (*J. Path. and Bact.*, 1913–14, **18**: 191–210); and Figs. 6 and 7 are from Sir Arthur Keith's Schorstein Lecture on this subject, "The fate of the bulbus cordis in the human heart," *Lancet*, Lond., Dec. 20, 1924, reproduced by kind permission of the authors and publishers.

Fig 1.—Order Teleostei. (Class Pisces.) Heart of angler (Lophius piscatorius).*

a. Dorsal surface showing sinus venosus opening into laterally expanded common auricle below, large thick-walled ventricle with spongy musculature in median line above, narrow bulbo-ventricular neck and bulbus cordis at extreme upper end giving off aortic arches cranially.

b. Ventral surface laid open to show common auriculo-ventricular orifice at lower end of ventricle in median line, single pair of semilunar valves at lower bulbar orifice. (Original drawings by W. W. Beattie and E. Shanly.)

Fig. 2.—Order Ganoidei. Heart of bony pike (Lepidosteus osseus).*

a. Bulbus cordis laid open to show rows of valves lining its lumen in different stages of development, the smaller, more rudimentary ones indicating retrogression incidental to the incipient spiral twisting that is taking place here.

b. Heart showing pyramidal-shaped ventricle below giving off slender elongated bulbus above, ending cranially in aortic arches. Auricle juts forward above and behind on either side of bulbus. (Drawings by W. W. Beattie and E. Shanly.)

Fig. 3.—Diagrams of the bulbus cordis of a, Elasmobranch fish; b, of Ceratodus; and c, Lepidosiren, the two latter being dipnoan fishes. In a there are four vertical rows of bulbar swellings or cusps, Nos. 1, 2, 3 and 4, those at the proximal extremities being numbered for comparison with b and c, 1, 2B, 3 and 4A, respectively. No spiral arrangement.

In diagram **b** the swellings are asymmetrically placed and form in the transverse portion (*B.C.e.*) a spiral valve (*Sp.v.*), where distal (*D*) and proximal (*P*) constrictions have occurred.

c. Distal ridges 2 and 4 have disappeared and 3 is a solid ridge while proximal ridges 1, 2B and 3 are merely vestigial. There remains only a spiral valve (*Sp.V.*), which begins above as distal ridge 1 and ends below in proximal ridge 4A. (From the article by Jane Robertson, Fig. 1 in her Plate XI.)

Fig. 4.—Order Elasmobranchii. Heart of skate (Raia erinacea).*

a. Ventral surface. The common ventricle curves definitely to the right and gives off the elongated conus lined by four horizontal rows of mucoid cusps arranged in vertical columns from its right upper end, while the common auriculo-ventricular orifice enters it at the left upper border. The auricle has ascended behind and above ventricle and pouches forward on either side.

b. Dorsal surface showing interior of common auricle expanded laterally with auriculo-ventricular orifice in lower left corner and sinus venosus below opening into its floor, between valvulae venosae a little to the right of the median line.

Fig. 5.—Order Urodela. (Class Amphibia.) Heart of mud-puppy (Necturus).*

a. Ventral view. The bulbus is a cordlike structure given off from right upper angle of pyramidal-shaped ventricle. Auricle to left and posteriorly above ventricle. B, bulbus; A, auricle; V, ventricle.

b. Dorsal view. Auricle shows beginning division of roof, receives orifice of sinus venosus below on right with entrance of pulmonary vein to left of this. *S.V.*, sinus venosus. (Drawings by W. W. Beattie and E. Shanly.)

Fig. 6.—Order Elasmobranchii. Heart of shark. Showing structure of muscular coats and primitive structure. (From a specimen in the London Hospital Museum, reported by Sir Arthur Keith, *l.c.* under Fig. 7.)

Fig. 7.—Diagram by Prof. Frazer of the human heart toward end of sixth week, showing transformation of bulbus and beginning division of aortic and pulmonary channels. A, right bulbar cushion; B, right cavity of bulb; C, aortic left posterior part of bulb; D, left bulbar cushion; E, interventricular septum; F, posterior and G, anterior endocardial cushions of auriculo-ventricular canal; H, mitral and J, tricuspid orifices; K, right and L, left ventricles; M, aortico-pulmonary septum with valve cushions. Arrows show directions of arterial and venous blood which will be divided later by fusion of right and left bulbar cushions (A and D) with right end of endocardial cushion G to left of tricuspid orifice. (Reproduced from Sir Arthur Keith's Schorstein Lecture, *Lancet*, Lond., Dec. 20, 1924, Figs. 1 and 16.)

* Specimen in the Cardiac Anomaly Collection of McGill University.

PLATE II. COMPARATIVE ANATOMY. FISH AND AMPHIBIAN HEART

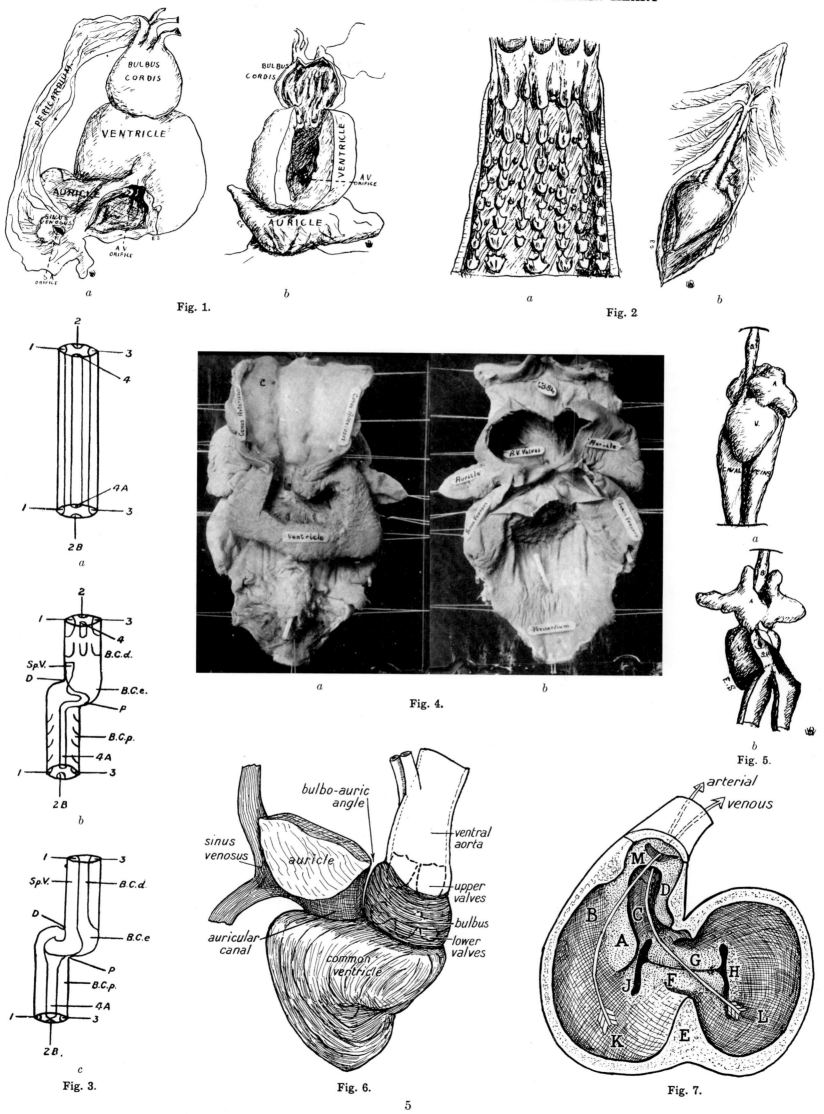

Fig. 1.

Fig. 2

Fig. 3.

Fig. 4.

Fig. 5.

Fig. 6.

Fig. 7.

5

PLATE III

COMPARATIVE ANATOMY (*Continued*). REPTILIAN HEART

A distinctive characteristic of the reptilian heart is the presence, in all orders, of a third arterial trunk, the reptilian right aorta, which, arising to the right of, and in close juxtaposition to, the abdominal viscera and lower extremities, coalesces some distance below the heart with a second large aorta, which transmits arterialized blood to the head and upper extremities (Fig. 4). The three vessels, each of which is supplied with a bicuspid semilunar valve, thus arise together from the base of the heart, encased usually in a tough fibrous sheath, and undergo at their origin a pronounced clockwise torsion from right to left upon each other, which is significant of the spiral arrangement of embryonic swellings in the primitive bulbus cordis, from fusion of which their three interarterial septa have been derived. The period of development at which these three arterial trunks are present together in the human embryonic heart is of extremely brief duration. That this stage does exist in it, however, is evident from the observation of embryologists and from the configuration of the normal right ventricle and also from the structure of various cardiac anomalies in which traces are plainly visible, fixed at the point of arrest. A comparative study of the successive stages in the evolution of these reptilian hearts as revealed in the turtle, python and crocodile throws a flood of light upon the complex processes that take place at the base of the organ in the sixth to eighth week of embryonic life, and conversely reveals, often with startling simplicity, the ontogenesis of many grave defects that may otherwise baffle analysis.

The first impetus to the study of these important interrelationships of cardiac defects as revealed in the comparative embryology of the vertebrate heart was given by the work of Roese (*Morphol. Jahrb.*, 1890, **16**: 2) and that of Greil on the development of the heart of *Lacerta agilis* (*l.c.* Pl. I, Fig. 3). There followed the fundamental contributions of Sir Arthur Keith, whose intensive studies upon persistence of the reptilian bulbus as the main etiological factor in pulmonary stenosis and other grave cardiac anomalies cast an entirely new light on the pathogenesis of these conditions (*J. Anat.*, Lond., 1905, **19**: 14; *Studies in Pathology*, Aberdeen, 1906; Hunterian Lectures, *Lancet*, Lond., 1909, **2**: 359, 433, 579; Schorstein Lecture, *ibid.*, 1924, **1**: 1267). There followed the valuable work of Jane Robertson upon the bulbar region of the fish and its bearing upon cardiac anomalies (*l.c.* Pl. II) and more recently Spitzer's brilliant theory (Pl. IV) of the part taken by delayed torsion with persistence of the "right" reptilian aorta in the causation of these conditions.

Acknowledgment is made of the kind assistance of Prof. J. S. Baxter in the revision of the descriptive text for this and the preceding plates (I and II) and in the preparation of the specimens shown in Figs. 2 and 3 opposite.

Fig. 1.—Order Chelonia. Heart of snapping turtle (Chelonia mydax). * a, ventral; b, dorsal surface. A three-chambered heart having two completely divided auricles, the right much larger than the left, which pouch forward above the large flattened common ventricle. The latter is incompletely divided dorso-ventrally by the bulbo-ventricular ridge (*B.V.R.*) into a smaller ventral chamber, giving off the pulmonary artery, and a large dorsal chamber, which gives off the right aorta posteriorly from its extreme upper right-hand corner and, just in front of this, the left systemic aorta. All three vessels are united at their base by a firm fibrous outer coat and each has a bicuspid valve. The dorsal ventricle is itself incompletely divided into shallow right and left cavities by an obliquely placed apical septum derived from the loose muscular trabeculae of its lower wall. That on its right side, known as the cavum venosum, receives the venous blood from the right auricle, while that on the left, the cavum arteriosum, receives the oxygenated blood from the left auricle but gives off no vessel. The auricular septum is entire and ends below in two large fleshy valvular cusps which act like paddles, propelling the venous blood from the cavum venosum into the pulmonary artery and left aorta, and the arterialized blood from the cavum arteriosum across the interventricular communication (*I.V.F.*) into the right aorta to be distributed to the vessels of the head and neck. This arrangement corresponds to that of a human embryonic heart about the end of fifth week. *A.C.*, anterior communication (bulbar septal defect); *Au.V.*, auriculo-ventricular cushions; *R.A.*, position of right auricle (removed in specimen); *G.C.*, gubernaculum cordis.

Fig. 2.—Diagram of reptilian heart. The dorsal ventricle is extended to right of ventral ventricle. Adapted from Walmsley (*Quain's Anatomy*, 1929, IV, III, p. 9). *B.V.R.*, bulbo-ventricular ridge; *R.V.*, ventral ventricle; *I.V.F.*, interventricular foramen; *C.Art.* and *C.Ven.*, cavum arteriosum and cavum venosum of dorsal ventricle; *P.A.*, pulmonary artery from ventral ventricle; right aorta from cavum venosum; left aorta from both ventral ventricle and cavum venosum of dorsal ventricle above bulbar septal defect (*A.C.*). (Diagram by A. C. Cheney, Medical Art Department, McGill University.)

Fig. 3.—Order Ophidia. Heart of water-snake (Matrix sitedon) in situ to show arrangement of great vessels. * The auricles have been pulled back to expose the origin of the three arterial trunks which emerge from the right upper angle of the ventricle as a single truncus. This is seen on close inspection to have two components twisted upon each other: the aortic stem, which divides after 0.75 cm. into the two systemic aortae, and the pulmonary artery, which arises anteriorly and to the left of this, and passes directly backward, emerging on its right side posteriorly and curving downward to reach the lungs in the abdomen. The two aortae curve upward on either side and then downward, the left supplying the abdominal viscera, and the right, which lies posteriorly, giving off the large branches to the head and upper extremities (right aortic arch). The two trunks unite some 3 cm. below the heart into a single trunk (double aortic arch). The right superior (*S.V.C.*) and inferior caval veins empty posteriorly into either end of the sinus venosus (*S.V.*), and the large left superior cava (*Lt.S.V.C.*) into the coronary sinus (*C.S.*).

(Drawing by A. G. Cheney from specimen No. 11393 presented by Prof. J. S. Baxter).

Fig. 4.—The same. Heart of python (P. molurus). * a, ventral, b, dorsal aspect. The heart shows a distinct advance on that of the turtle in that torsion of the great trunks is increased and the apical septum dividing the dorsal ventricle into its two cava (see Fig. 2) is considerably higher and the interventricular foramen (*I.V.F.*) smaller, while the bulbo-ventricular ridge is likewise more developed, forming a distinct floor for the ventral ventricle and reducing the bulbar septal defect to a linear slit (*AC*). The effect is that of a heart with three ventricles and two completely divided auricles. In the lower part of the floor of the ventral ventricle is a small round communication (*PC*) in its trabeculae with the cavum arteriosum of the dorsal ventricle, permitting of an arterial-venous or venous-arterial shunt between these two chambers. The two large valvular flaps attached on either border of the lower end of the auricular septum perform their paddle-like action, sending the venous blood from the cavum venosum toward the pulmonary artery and left aorta (*L.Ao.*) and thereafter the arterialized blood from the cavum arteriosum through the interventricular foramen (*I.V.F.*) into the right aorta, (*R.Ao*). *R.AV* and *L.AV*, right and left venous ostia, *SVC*, superior, *IVC*, inferior vena cava. (Drawing by W. W. Beattie and E. Shanly.)

Fig. 5.—Order Crocodilia. Heart of crocodile (Alligator mississippiensis). * This organ is of great interest because it reveals the final stages in closure of the communications that exist between the chambers in the turtle and python heart and thus sheds light upon the completion of the mammalian interventricular septum. This has been accomplished by the growth downward of a muscular tongue of tissue between the right and left aortae (lower border of aortic septum) and the further torsion of the great trunks and bulbar portion of the heart upon each other so that this process meets and finally fuses with the left border of the right auriculo-ventricular orifice. Thus the right aorta is placed in the now completely separated cavum arteriosum of the dorsal ventricle, while the pulmonary artery and left aorta remain in the ventral ventricle, which has now come to contain also the cavum venosum of the dorsal chamber. The only communication between the two circulations that remains is a secondary aperture, the *foramen Panizzae*, which has developed in the contiguous sinuses of Valsalva of the right and left aortae where these cross each other and which permits arterialized blood from the right aorta to flow at intervals into the left aortic (venous) trunk. The spiral twisting that has taken place in the separation of the ventricles is plainly visible in the convex floor of the ventral ventricle and in the twisted relations of the great trunks. (From a specimen in the collection of the late Prof. G. S. Huntington. Reproduced from the article by M. E. Abbott in *Contributions to Medical and Biological Research*, dedicated to Sir William Osler, 1919, Fig. 5, Paul B. Hoeber, New York.)

Fig. 6.—The aortic arches and their transformations (after Rathke). 1. Ceratodus. 2. Salamander. 3. Triton. 4. Frog. 5. Lizard. 6. Bird. 7. Mammal. (Republished by permission from the article by H. A. Harris, *J. Anat.*, Lond., 1922, **57**: Part I, 85.)

* Specimen in the Cardiac Anomaly Collection of McGill University.

PLATE III. COMPARATIVE ANATOMY (*Continued*). THE REPTILIAN HEART

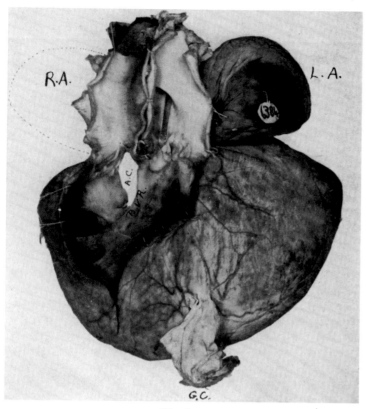

Fig. 1a.

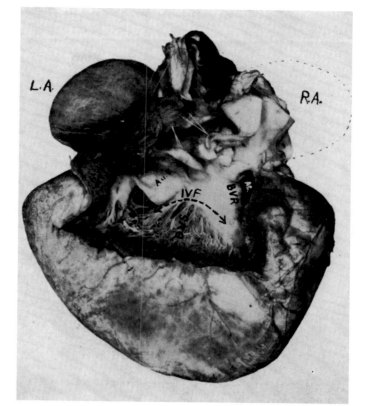

Fig. 1b.

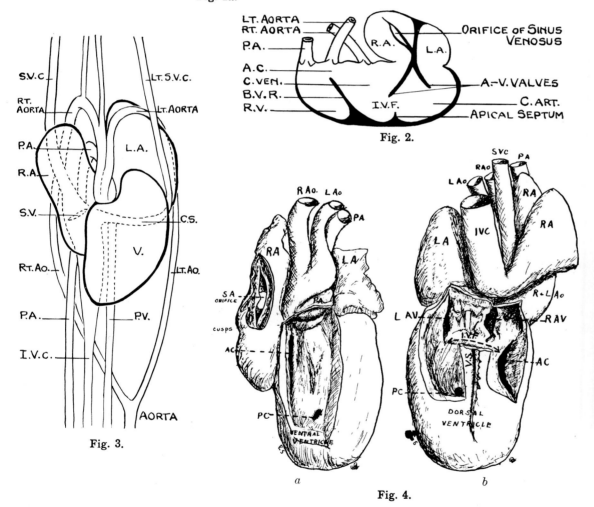

LT. AORTA		
RT. AORTA		ORIFICE OF SINUS
P.A.	R.A. L.A.	VENOSUS
A.C.		
C. VEN.		A-V. VALVES
B.V.R.		C. ART.
R.V.	I.V.F.	APICAL SEPTUM

Fig. 2.

Fig. 3.

Fig. 4.

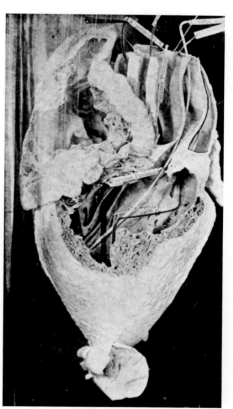

Fig. 5.

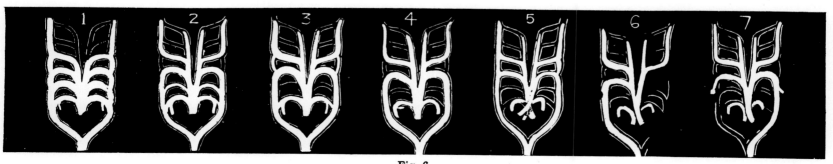

Fig. 6.

PLATE IV

INCOMPLETE TORSION IN THE CAUSATION OF CARDIAC DEFECTS (SPITZER'S THEORY)

In 1875, Carl von Rokitansky published his epoch-making work on the pathogenesis of cardiac septal defects. Based on an exact morphological study of his own great collection carried out in the light of the then new science of embryology, the facts elicited by him and his brilliant deductions therefrom may be said to have unlocked the door for the more exact scientific investigation of this great subject and definitely placed the origin of these obscure conditions in the very early weeks of embryonic life. The curious manner in which the graver cardiac anomalies mirror the hearts of the lower vertebrate orders had been commented upon ever since the time of Meckel (1812) and the correlation of these in recent years with their phylogenetic prototypes in the stage of embryonic life at which arrest had occurred has greatly clarified our understanding of these obscure conditions. The fundamental contribution of Sir Arthur Keith upon the persistence of the reptilian bulbus in the causation of pulmonary stenosis and allied anomalies (*l.c.* Pl. II and III) marks an important milestone on the line of advance in this respect and since then other workers in the same field of anatomical research have added their quota to our knowledge.

It has remained, however, for Prof. Alexander Spitzer of Vienna, upon whom the mantle of Rokitansky's genius seems to have fallen in our own generation, to originate a teleological theory of startling simplicity, based upon the indisputable evidence of vestigial remains in the right ventricle which link the human heart with the reptilian in a common ancestry. This theory has revolutionized many of our ideas on the ontogenesis of these defects and has supplied the most satisfactory explanation as yet available of those bizarre conditions of transposed great vessels and inverted ventricles that have seemed to contradict every known principle of development or evolution. Briefly described, it ascribes such anomalies to the arrest or delay of the clockwise torsion that normally takes place in the growth of the primitive embryonic heart between its fixed arterial and venous ends during the process of septation, thus leading to an apparently counter-clockwise shunting of the parts with resultant reopening of the channel of the reptilian right aorta and obliteration of the left ventricular vessel. Anatomical proof of the latter curious fact is supplied by the confirmation of the right ventricle in which the trabecula septomarginalis or moderator band is homologous (as observed by Tandler) with the septum between the right aorta and pulmonary artery in the reptilian heart; that portion of the ventricle lying between the "anterior tricuspid ledge" of the latter and the crista supraventricularis being identified as the "outflow channel" of the "right reptilian aorta," which is closed in the normal human heart by the clockwise torsion of the bulbo-ventricular end of the primitive cardiac tube. An additional very suggestive point is seen in the persistence of the bicuspid pulmonary valve (normal in reptiles) in the developmental form of pulmonary stenosis. Further explanation of this very intriguing and suggestive theory is to be sought in Prof. Spitzer's own meticulously detailed and beautifully worked out monograph (reference under Fig. 3) or may be gathered from the writer's summary (*Nelson's Loose-leaf Med.*, 1932, **2**: 214–218), where the figures opposite also appear.

Fig. 1.—Spitzer's diagrams showing relationship of the semilunar cusps, bulbar swellings and septa in the reptilian and normal human heart, and in a malformed human heart with bicuspid pulmonary valve.

A. Reptilian heart. Here there are three trunks, the primary septum aortico-pulmonale (*S.ao.p.I*) and the septum aorticum (*S.ao.*) together forming the septum between the pulmonary artery and left aorta, but dividing anteriorly to enclose the right aorta (*rt.ao.*). Each vessel has only two cusps as the primary septum aortico-pulmonale does not reach the valvular part of the bulbar swelling.

B. Normal human heart. The septum aorticum has united throughout with the primary septum aortico-pulmonale to form the secondary septum aortico-pulmonale. The right aorta has disappeared. Only two great vessels exist and each has three cusps.

C. Malformed heart with pulmonary stenosis and bicuspid pulmonary valve. The aortic septum has disappeared and the left aorta has become obliterated or fused with the right aorta. Only one large vessel (the right reptilian aorta) exists on the right anteriorly. The pulmonary orifice is smaller and has only two cusps because the primary aortico-pulmonary septum does not meet the valvular part of the bulbar swelling (III).

I, II, III, IV, distal bulbar swellings; *A, B, C*, proximal bulbar swellings extended into bulbar region; *Iv., IIv., IIIv., IVv.*, valvular parts of distal bulbar region; *Is., IIs.*, septal parts of the distal bulbar region; *S.Vt.*, septum ventriculorum; *P*, pulmonary artery.

Fig. 2.—Heart in a case of persistence of the right ventricular aorta (Spitzer's Type II) with rudimentary interventricular septum (cor biatriatum triloculare) and stenosed and bicuspid pulmonary valve. (Note the cleft (*N*) marking the orifice of the rudimentary conus of the obliterated left ventricular aorta.) *C*, the hypertrophied crista supraventricularis (aortico-pulmonary septum); *S*, upper border of rudimentary interventricular septum which separates the stenosed pulmonary ostium anteriorly from the deep niche or cleft (*N*), which is the rudimentary conus of the obliterated left ventricular aorta. Behind and to the left of this niche is the aortic segment of the mitral valve. *T*, trabecula septomarginalis.

From a boy aged 5 with extreme cyanosis and clubbing. (Reported by Mautner and Löwy under title "Transposition der Aorta oder Persistenz der rechtskammerigen Aorta," *Virch. Arch.*, 1931, **229**: 337.)

Fig. 3.—Diagrams showing division of the ventricles and relative positions of the arterial ostia in the normal heart and in the different types of transposition of the great trunks as conceived in Spitzer's phylogenetic theory of persistent right reptilian aorta and formation of a septum spurium in the right ventricle.

a. Normal human heart. *A.P.*, pulmonary artery; *Ao.*, normal (left ventricular) aorta; *Ao. rt.*, obliterated conus of right aorta; *Mi.* and *Tric.*, mitral and tricuspid valves; *va., vp.* and *vm.*, anterior, posterior and median tricuspid cusps; *cr.*, crista supraventricularis; *as.* and *s.p.*, anterior and posterior part of interventricular septum.

b. Type I of transposition: "*reitende*" aorta (fusion of both aortic trunks).

c. Type II, "simple" transposition (aorta from right ventricle).

d. Type III, "crossed" transposition, aorta arising from the right and the pulmonary from the left ventricle.

e. Type IV, "mixed" transposition, the pulmonary artery and both auriculo-ventricular ostia in a common chamber and aorta arising transposed from small right ventricle. *a.Tr.r.*, anterior tricuspid ridge; *A.Sr.* and *p.S.r.*, anterior and posterior septal ridges; *a.P.Mi.* and *P.P.Mi.*, anterior and posterior papillary muscles of mitral valve; *p.p.Tr.*, posterior papillary muscle of tricuspid. (From A. L. Spitzer, "Über den Bauplan des normalen und missbildeten Herzens," *Virch. Arch.*, 1923, **243**: 81–272. Diagrams adapted by J. Fleury.)

Fig. 4.—Diagrams illustrating a case of "crossed" transposition (Spitzer's Type III, aorta in right ventricle, pulmonary artery in left ventricle), showing plan of base of ventricles seen from above (after Spitzer).

A. In the normal mammalian heart. *S.vt.*, septum ventriculorum; *Cr. + Tsm.*, crista supraventricularis + trabecula septomarginalis; *Co.rt.Ao.*, blind ending of rudimentary conus of right ventricular aorta; *Mi., Tri.*, mitral and tricuspid orifices.

B. In the anomalous heart described showing transposed aorta. *Ao [rt.Ao]*, the transposed (right reptilian) aorta; *Cr.*, the markedly hypertrophied crista aortico-pulmonaris (supraventricularis), forming spurious ventricular septum; *a.S.vt.*, the atrophic true anterior interventricular septum; and *Co.lt.Ao*, blind ending of the left ventricular aorta; *a.T.l.* anterior tricuspid ledge. (By P. Freudenthal, *Virch. Arch.*, 1927–28, **226**: 640.)

Fig. 5.—Heart showing niche of the obliterated right aorta in normal right ventricle. This ventricle laid open to show its interior which is of normal configuration except that the crista supraventricularis is heavily developed, thus bringing into prominence a deep crevice lying posteriorly between it and the infundibular tricuspid segment. This is the niche and outflow tract of the obliterated right aorta.

From an infant dying three hours after birth. The ventricular septum was entire and the foramen ovale and ductus arteriosus were widely patent, the pulmonary artery forming the descending aorta through the latter channel. The heart lay entirely in the right thorax. Multiple somatic anomalies. (From a specimen in the possession of L. Minor Blackford, Atlanta, Ga., kindly supplied for illustration of this point in this Atlas. Drawing by A. C. Cheney, Medical Art Department, McGill University.)

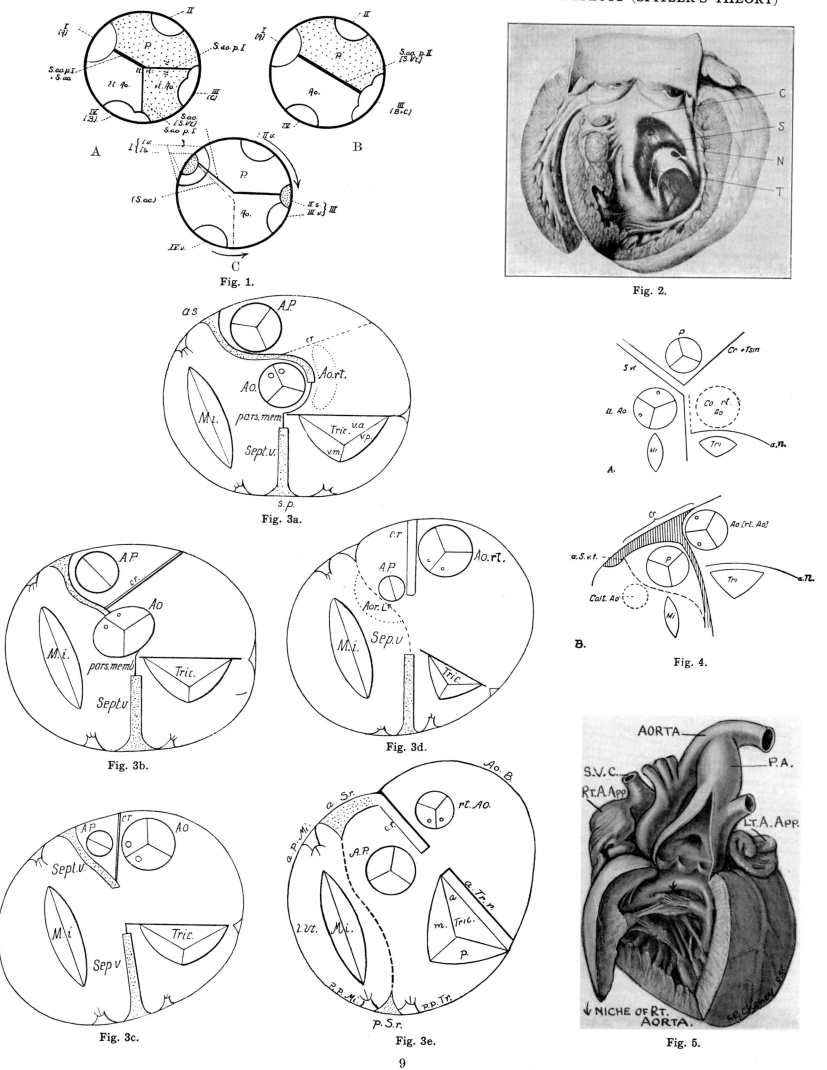

Fig. 1.

Fig. 2.

Fig. 3a.

Fig. 4.

Fig. 3b.

Fig. 3d.

Fig. 3c.

Fig. 3e.

Fig. 5.

PART II
CLINICAL CLASSIFICATION OF CONGENITAL CARDIAC DISEASE

GROUP I. No Abnormal Communication (Acyanotic Group)

GROUP II. Cases of Arterial-Venous Shunt with Terminal Reversal of Flow (Cyanose Tardive)

GROUP III. Cases of Permanent Venous-Arterial Shunt and Retardation of Flow (Cyanotic Group)

PLATE V

THE CLINICAL CLASSIFICATION OF CARDIAC DEFECTS. ILLUSTRATIVE DIAGRAMS

The clinical significance of cardiac anomalies depends upon the pathological physiology of the altered circulation as induced by the defect. This may be of the nature of a simple mechanical obstruction which leads directly to undue strain at exposed points, but in which there is *no abnormal communication* between the systemic and pulmonary circulations and therefore no cause for cyanosis is present (Group I; Fig. 1). Or, secondly, an anomalous aperture may exist in the form of a *localized, uncomplicated* defect in the cardiac or aortic septa, through which, so long as the pressure remains physiologically higher on the left or systemic side, oxygenated blood passes into the pulmonary circulation. An *arterial-venous shunt* exists, until pathological conditions supervene, raising the pressure on the right side of the defect; then the direction of the shunt will be reversed and venous blood will flow into the arterial stream (*cyanose tardive*) (Group II; Fig. 2). Thirdly, if such a localized defect be complicated by associated anomalies which permanently raise the pressure on the venous side; or if one or more of the cardio-vascular septa be entirely absent; or if the great trunks arise transposed from reversed ventricles (Figs. 3*a*, *b*, *c*), a *permanent venous-arterial shunt* will result with development of capillary changes and a persistent *morbus coeruleus*. In addition, a small group must be recognized in which, without any abnormal communication between the two circulations, a mechanical obstruction to the return of venous blood to the right heart exists, leading to *retardation of flow* in the capillaries, and *persistent cyanosis from capillary stasis* and *increased deoxygenation* at the periphery (Group III (*b*) below).

On the basis of the above considerations the following classification has been formulated of cardiac anomalies of clinical significance.

I. *Acyanotic group.* Cases in which no *abnormal communication* exists between the two circulations but in which the anomaly is liable to become the seat of strain.

II. *Cyanose tardive group.* Cases of arterial-venous shunt with possible *transient* or *terminal* reversal of flow.

III. *Cyanotic group.* (*a*) Cases of *permanent arterial-venous shunt*, with resultant capillary changes. (*b*) Cases of *simple retardation of flow*, (right-sided valvular lesions with all foetal passages closed). Pl. XVII.

Acknowledgment. The large series of diagrams illustrating the course of the circulation in the different individual defects which are used as key features heading Plates XIII to XV (Group II) and Plates XVIII to XXIV (Group III) were drawn by Garnet Jex of the Medical Art Department of the Army Medical Museum, Washington, D. C., for illustration of the article by M. E. Abbott and W. T. Dawson on "The Clinical Classification of Congenital Cardiac Disease" which appeared in *International Clinics*, 1924, IV, Ser. **34**: 155; and the figures opposite were drawn by P. Larivière of the Medical Art Department of McGill University after the diagrams by Louis Gross, and appeared in the writer's article on this subject, published, *ibid.*, 1934, III, Ser. **44**: 15. The writer's thanks are expressed to both sources and to the J. B. Lippincott Company, publishers, for kind permission to reproduce these very useful diagrams here. Figures 1*a*, 1*c* and 2*b* are reproduced from the writer's monograph in Osler's *Modern Medicine*, 3d ed., by permission of Lea and Febiger, publisher.

For additional references on this subject see the writer's articles in *Osler's Mod. Med.*, 1927, **4**: 653–657; *Lancet*, Lond., July 27, 1929; *Brit. Med. J.*, Dec. 31, 1932; and *Nelson's Loose-leaf Med.*, 1932, **4**: 226–229. Also D. C. Muir and J. W. Brown, "Congenital heart disease," *Brit. Med. J.*, 1935, **1**: 966; and "Clinical Classification of Congenital Cardiovascular Disease," in *Heart Disease* by Paul D. White, 1931, 310–313, The Macmillan Company, New York.

Fig. 1.—**Diagram showing the course of the circulation under normal conditions and in cardiac anomalies** in which there is **no abnormal communication** between the two circulations, with examples of defects which fall under this category (Group I).

a. Right aortic arch with total suppression of left.* The ligamentum arteriosum crosses behind the trachea and oesophagus to be attached to the right arch, thus encircling these viscera in a vascular ring, a condition which is liable to give rise to pressure symptoms of dysphagia and dyspnoea. From a woman aged 61, dying of intestinal obstruction. (Drawing by Prof. J. G. Adami of specimen No. 15.11.[1] Reported by M. E. Abbott in *Osler's Mod. Med.*, 1927, **4**: 791, Fig. 93. Reprinted on Plate VI, Fig. 6.)

b. The diagram illustrating this group. *P.V.R.*, pulmonary venous reservoir; *S.V.R.*, systemic venous reservoir; *S.V.C.*, superior vena cava; *I.V.C.*, inferior vena cava; *C.*, conus of right ventricle; *A.*, aorta and aortic vestibule; *P.A.*, pulmonary artery; *R.A.*, *R.V.*, right auricle and ventricle; *L.A.*, *L.V.*, left auricle and ventricle.

c. Anomalous origin of left coronary from pulmonary artery.* Heart showing cirsoid dilatations and sacculation of both coronaries, due to the blood entering the anastomotic branches of each under different pressures and producing the effect of an arterio-venous aneurysm. *A*, vascular loop the size of a crabapple just beyond the origin of the right coronary, giving off its descending branches; *B*, dilated transverse branch of the same; *C*, circumflex and *D*, descending branches of the left coronary.

From a woman aged 60 who died accidentally. The heart was hypertrophied and the seat of replacement fibrosis and fatty changes. (Drawing by Prof. J. G. Adami from specimen No. 15.145.[1] Reported by M. E. Abbott, *ibid.*, 795, Fig. 94.)

Fig. 2.—**Diagrams of the circulation in cases of localized uncomplicated cardiac septal defect leading to an arterial-venous shunt with reversal of flow.** With example of a defect falling under this category (Group II Lettering as in Fig. 1*b* (cf. Pl. XIII–XV).

a. Circulation under physiological conditions in which the pressure is normally higher in the left ventricle causing the shunt to pass from left to right through the defect as occurs in compensated septal defects.

b. Heart showing a large defect at the lower part of the interauricular septum (persistent ostium primum) illustrating this type of anomaly. Associated with *double mitral orifice*, cleavage of the anterior segment of the mitral valve, patent foramen ovale and bifid apex. Accidental findings in a child of 5 years. (Reported by M. E. Abbott, *ibid.*, 759, Fig. 88.)

c. Circulation when pathological conditions supervene, causing a relative rise of pressure in the right chambers or in the pulmonary circulation, producing a reversal of flow from right to left through the defect (indicated by dotted arrow) and mixture of venous blood with the arterial stream (cyanose tardive).

Fig. 3.—**Diagrams of the circulation in cases of permanent venousarterial shunt** (congenital cyanosis), Group III. A black arrow is passed through the patent foramen ovale. *P.D.A.*, patent ductus. Other lettering as in Fig. 1*b*.

a. Circulation in the tetralogy of Fallot (defect at base of interventricular septum with dextroposition of aorta and pulmonary stenosis), in which venous blood passes from right to left through the defect and the pressure is also raised in the systemic capillaries (cf. Pl. XIX).

b. In complete absence of the interventricular septum (cor triloculare biatriatum) showing free admixture of venous and arterial streams in the common ventricle (cf. Pl. XXI).

c. In complete transposition of great trunks with ventricular septum closed, foramen ovale and ductus arteriosus patent. Note that the sole pathway for the aerated blood from the lungs is through the foramen ovale into the transposed aorta (cf. Pl. XXIII).

* Specimen in the Cardiac Anomaly Collection of McGill University.

(*Continued on page* 14.)

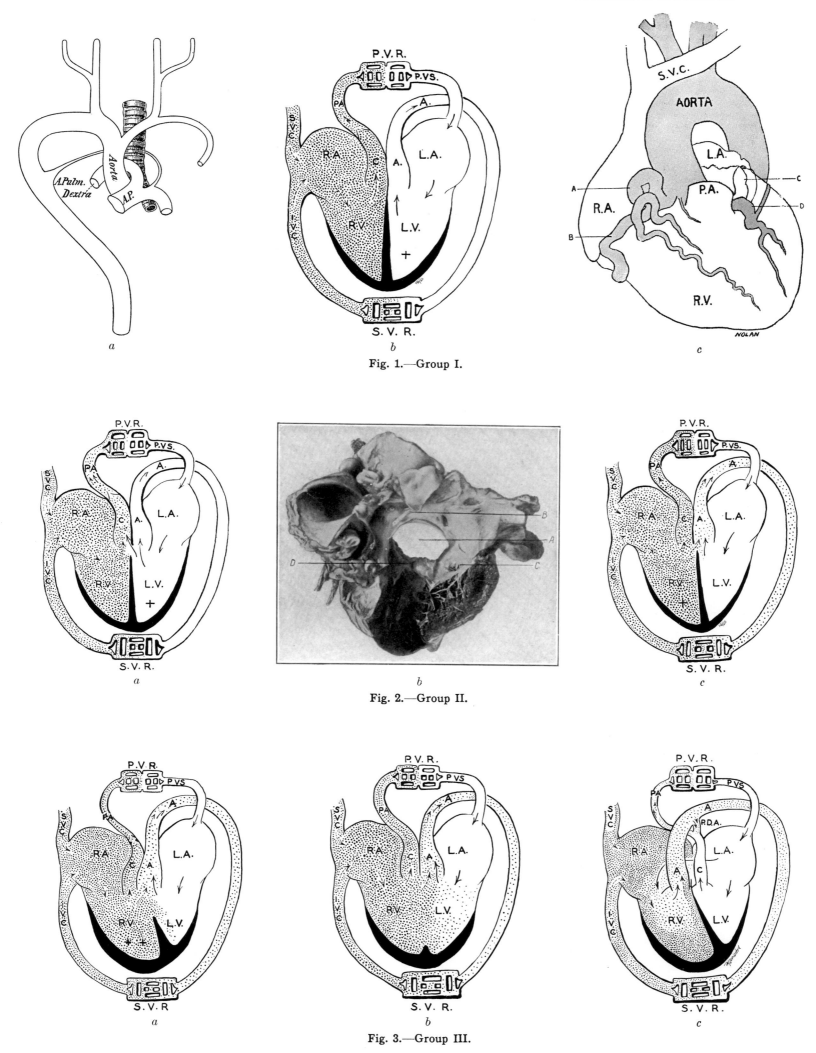

Fig. 1.—Group I.

Fig. 2.—Group II.

Fig. 3.—Group III.

13

PLATE V (*Continued*)

DETAILS OF FOREGOING CLASSIFICATION

A. Cardiac Defects of Clinical Significance

Note: In the list below the figures given showing relative incidence and duration of life in the various defects are drawn from the writer's chart of 1000 cases analyzed (see pp. 60–61), the total number of cases of the individual lesion being taken from the last column, and the highest and average age, etc., in the number of cases listed as the primary lesion from the first three columns.

I. *Acyanotic group. Left-sided lesions with no abnormal communication between the two circulations.* Such are: pericardial defect, 31 cases (average age in 28 cases classed as primary lesion 42 years, highest 75); congenital so-called idiopathic hypertrophy, 17 cases (average in 15 cases 4 months, highest 4 years); congenital heart block, 4 cases (average in 3 cases 7 years, highest 20); anomalous septa in auricles, 30 cases (average in 12 cases 22⅖ years, highest 58); congenital aortic and mitral stenosis, 34 cases (average in 17 cases 3 years, highest 27); bicuspid aortic valve, 78 cases (average in 32 cases 33 years, highest 68); bicuspid pulmonary valve, 31 cases (age in 1 case classed as primary lesion 20); supernumerary aortic cusps, 4 cases (average in 2 cases 36 years, highest 41); supernumerary pulmonary cusps, 12 cases (average in 8 cases 36 years, highest 80); double mitral orifice, 10 cases (average in 8 cases 37 years, highest 71); pulmonary dilatation, 9 cases (average in 6 cases 14 years, highest 59); coarctation of aorta of adult type, 105 cases (average in 70 cases 33 years, highest 92—Reynaud's case); hypoplasia of aorta (average in 2 cases listed 19 years); double and right aortic arch, 40 cases (average in 19 cases 32½ years, highest 87); left coronary from pulmonary artery, 10 cases (average in 8 cases 36 years, highest 61); congenital arterio-venous aneurysm, 8 cases (average in 6 cases 21 years, highest 35) congenital rhabdomyoma, 17 cases (highest age 20 years).

II. *Cases of arterial-venous shunt with possible transient or terminal reversal of flow (cyanose tardive).* (1) Patent ductus arteriosus, 242 cases (average in 92 cases 24 years, highest 56); Paul D. White's case. (2) Persistent patency of foramen ovale, 290 cases (average in 40 cases 29 years, highest 70); defect at upper part of interauricular septum, 19 cases (average in 10 cases 34 years, highest 64); defect in the lower part of the interauricular septum, 36 cases (average in 18 cases 19 years, highest 46); premature closure of foramen ovale, 4 cases (average in 3 cases 18 hours). (3) Localized defects of the interventricular septum, *maladie de Roger*, 257 cases (average in 50 cases 14½ years, highest 49); elsewhere or multiple, 28 cases (average in 5 cases 23 years, highest 79—Weiss's case); aneurysm of pars membranacea, 16 cases (average in 7 cases 42 years, highest 60). (4) Defects of aortic septum: congenital aneurysm of aortic sinus of Valsalva (average in 12 cases 28 years, highest 53); communication between aorta and pulmonary artery (average in 10 cases 14 years, highest 48).

III. *Cyanotic group.* Lesions or combinations of lesions arranged below in the order of increasing depth of cyanosis and lessened duration of life.

(a) *Right-sided valvular lesions with foetal passages closed* and *in* which there are stasis and increased deoxygenation in the capillaries, leading to *moderate cyanosis* with clubbing of late appearance: pulmonary stenosis with closed septa, 11 cases (average in 9 cases 10½ years, highest 45—Hebb's case); congenital tricuspid stenosis with closed septa, average age in 2 cases listed 22 years.

(b) *Cases of permanent venous-arterial shunt* with resultant capillary changes. Cardiovascular septal defects complicated by right-sided valvular lesions, complete absence of cardiac or arterial septa, "complete" or "partial" transposition of great trunks, isolated congenital dextrocardia.

Moderate cyanosis. Pulmonary stenosis with closed ventricular septum but patent foramen ovale, 20 cases (average in 16 cases 18 years, highest 57—case by Lallemand); tricuspid atresia with defective auricular septum and transposition of great trunks (one case only, recorded by Hedinger in 1915, lived 56 years); dextroposition of aorta with defect at base of ventricular septum *without* pulmonary stenosis, 121 cases (average in 10 cases 13 years, highest 45 years); complete absence of interventricular septum (cor biatriatum triloculare), 27 cases (highest age 35—case by Mann); common auriculo-ventricular ostium, 14 cases (average in 10 cases 1½ months, highest 4¾ years).

Marked cyanosis. Pulmonary stenosis with defect of interventricular septum, 20 cases (average in 85 cases 14¼ years, highest 59 years 9 months—White's musician); pulmonary atresia with defect of interventricular septum, 49 cases (average in 30 cases 6¼ years, highest 30—Bach's case); persistent truncus, complete defect of aortic septum, 34 cases (average in 21 cases 4⅛ years, highest 25—Zimmerman's case); complete transposition of great arterial trunks with defect of interventricular septum, 36 cases (average age in 16 other cases 1½ years, highest 16—case by Keith); cor biloculare with transposition of great trunks (1 case was reported by Rudolf, aged 16 years; (*vide infra*).

Extreme cyanosis. Morbus coeruleus from birth. Transposition of great trunks with *closed* ventricular septum, ductus arteriosus and foramen ovale patent, 38 cases (average age in 31 other cases was 1¾ months, highest age reached was 11 years—case of Emanuel); pulmonary atresia with *closed* interventricular septum, ductus arteriosus and foramen ovale patent (highest age in a patient reported by Costa was 20 years, average age in 9 others 2¼ months); tricuspid atresia, 25 cases (Hedinger's case with transposition reached 56, average age of 15 other cases 5 months); cor biloculare, 14 cases (1 case by Wood and Williams attained 15 years and 1 by Rudolf with transposition 16 years, average age in 7 other cases 5½ weeks); mitral atresia, 13 cases (highest age 3½ years—Blackmore, average in 4 other cases 5 weeks); aortic atresia, 14 cases (average in 12 cases 4 days, highest 15 weeks—case by Simmons).

B. Cases of No Clinical Significance

Diverticulum of pericardium, bifid apex of heart, diverticulum of heart, acardia and ectopia cordis pectoralis (as being non-viable), true (mirror-picture) dextrocardia in complete situs inversus are conditions that come under this heading. Such cases are not figured here.

GENERAL REFERENCES

Abbott, Maude E., "Congenital cardiac disease," monograph in Osler and McCrae's *System of Modern Medicine*, 1st ed., 1908, **4**: 323–425; 2d ed., 1915, **4**: 323–448; 3d ed., 1927, **4**: 612–812. *Also:* "The treatment of congenital cardiac disease," in Blumer-Billings-Forschheimer's *System of Therapeutics*, D. Appleton Company, 1924, 302–362. *Also:* "The diagnosis of congenital cardiac disease" in *Blumer's Bedside Diagnosis*, W. B. Saunders Company, 1928, **2**: 357–574. *Also:* "Congenital heart disease," in *Nelson's Loose-leaf Medicine*, Thomas Nelson & Sons, 1932, **4**, 207–321.

Fleury, J., "Les affections congènitales, in Encyclopèdie Medico-chirurgicale, 1934, **12**.

Herzheimer, G., Missbildungen des Herzens und der Gefässe, in *Schwalbe's Missbildungen*, 1910, Part III, 339.

Humphry, L., "Congenital diseases of the heart," in Allbutt's *System of Medicine*, 1909, **6**, 276.

Laubry, C., and C. Pezzi, *Traité des maladies congènitales du coeur*, J. B. Baillière et fils, Paris, 1921.

Mönckeberg-Bonn, J. G., "Die Missbildungen des Herzens," *Henke u. Lubarsch Handbuch*, 1924, II.

Muir D. C. and J. W. Brown, Congenital Heart Disease, *Brit. Med. J.*, 1935, **1**, 1966.

Osler, W., "Congenital affections of the heart," in *Keating's Cyclop. Dis Child.*, 1889, **2**, 747.

Peacock, T. B., *On Malformations of the Human Heart with Original Cases*, London, 1858; 2d ed., 1866.

Thérémin, *Études congènitales du coeur*, St. Petersburg, 1895.

Thomson, J., "Congenital heart disease," *Oxford Medicine*, 1920, **2**, 371.

Thorel, In *Lubarsch-Ostertag's Ergebnisse*, 1903, Ch. II, p. 585; 1910, Ch. I, p. 585; 1910, Ch. II, p. 268.

Vierordt, H., "Die augeborenen Herzkrankheiten," in *Nothnagel's System*, 1898, **15**, 244.

White, Paul D., On cardiac anomalies in Chap. XII of his *Heart Disease*, The MacMillan Co., 2nd ed. 1936.

GROUP I
NO ABNORMAL COMMUNICATION
(ACYANOTIC GROUP)

PLATE VI

ANOMALIES OF THE AORTIC ARCH AND ITS BRANCHES

The evanescent character of the six pairs of embryonic arches, which replace each other in rapid transition as the heart ascends in the thorax, supplies the basis for a well-recognized series of anomalies in which arrest has occurred at a point that is commonly mirrored in the hearts of the lower orders of vertebrates (see Pl. III, Fig. 6 and Congdon, *Amer. J. Anat.*, 1926, **37**: 499). The only embryonic arches that persist in their entirety in the normal human heart are the fourth left, which becomes the definitive aorta, and the third pair (carotid), while the right fourth arch is normally suppressed in part, its cephalic portion only persisting as the innominate. Persistence may occur of both fourth arches in their entire length, constituting a *double aortic arch* in which (*a*) *both trunks may be of full caliber* as in Figs. 4 and 5 opposite, or (*b*) *the left member of the pair may be stenosed or obliterated* usually in the region of the foetal isthmus as in Arkin's case (Fig. 2). Again, a *right aortic arch* may occur (*a*) with total suppression of the left (Fig. 6) or (*b*) the caudal or distal portion of the latter may, and usually does, coexist (*right aortic arch with persistent left root*). Finally, if suppression of the right or left fourth arch has occurred before the ascent of the subclavians, one of the latter will arise from the descending arch or thoracic aorta, the right subclavian from a persistent right root (Fig. 8), or the left subclavian from a left root or from the ductus or pulmonary artery (Fig. 7). The clinical significance of all these cases, except the anomalous left subclavian, lies in the fact that a vascular ring is formed encircling and sometimes compressing the trachea and oesophagus with resultant dysphagia and dyspnoea. A correct diagnosis can usually be made by barium-x-ray investigation (Figs. 1, 3, 4). Anomalous origin of the right pulmonary from the innominate (Fig. 9) is a rare condition, explained by the author of the case reported below (Fig. 9) as a substitution of the right fifth arch.

In this connection see the valuable illustrated monograph by Williams Evans of the Cardiac Department of the London Hospital entitled "The Course of the Oesophagus in Health and in Disease of the Heart and Great Vessels," just published under the *British Medical Research Council, Special Report Ser. No. 208*, London, 1936.

Fig. 1.—Roentgenogram after barium meal in antero-posterior diameter from a case of right aortic arch. The course of the oesophagus is visualized and has been outlined in white and shows a characteristic sharp curve with convexity to the left and behind this on the right a retro-oesophageal shadow of the right aorta. From a boy, aged 10, with multiple associated anomalies. (Case of L. M. Blackford, *Amer. J. Dis. Child.*, 1932, **44**: 823).

Fig. 2.—Double aortic arch with atresia of left isthmus. The aorta arises by a broad base and arches up to the right and posteriorly giving off a large left innominate and thereafter the right carotid and subclavian. The left subclavian is attached near its origin by a short fibrous cord (obliterated isthmus) to a diverticulum which projects toward it from the descending arch (left aortic root), the whole forming a vascular ring encircling the trachea and oesophagus. A long ligamentum arteriosum attached the atresic isthmus to the left pulmonary artery. From a man aged 50, dying of periarteritis nodosa. Diagnosis made before death by x-ray which showed in right oblique diameter the right aortic knob behind the trachea and within this the round shadow of the left aortic root. (From the article by A. Arkin, *Wien. Arch. f. inn. Med.*, 1926, **12**: 385, Case 1, Pl. XVI, Fig. 1.)

Fig. 3.—Orthodiagraph of right aortic arch after barium meal in right oblique diameter. Note curve forward of oesophagus and right aortic knob behind this, which are diagnostic. *tra.*, trachea; *oes.*, oesophagus; *ao. k.*, aortic knob. (Arkin's Case 2, *ibid.*, Pl. XIV, Fig. 2.)

Fig. 4.—Antero-posterior roentgenogram after barium meal in a case of double aortic arch with total persistence of left arch. Note that the aortic shadow at the level of the third and fourth dorsal vertebrae is uniformly constricted on all sides and is *not deflected to the left* as in simple right aortic arch (cf. Fig. 1) or in double aortic arch with atresic isthmus (Arkin's Case 1), a diagnostic point. Female, aged 5 months with noisy inspiration and respiratory distress, death from bronchopneumonia. (From the article by C. E. Snelling and I. H. Erb, *Arch. Dis. Child.*, 1933, **8**: 401.)

Fig. 5.—Double aortic arch with total persistence of left arch which is of good caliber and completely pervious. Classic type. The ascending aorta, which is wider than normal, arches upward and backward on the right and splits at its convexity into two transverse branches of which the larger lies above and posteriorly and gives off the right subclavian and carotid while the smaller lies in front and anteriorly and gives off the two left trunks, the two arches enclosing an ovoid cleft 1.6 by 3 cm. long, beyond which they unite to form the large descending left arch 8 cm. in circumference. The trachea and oesophagus lie in the cleft and are flattened but not constricted. An accidental finding in a Greek man, aged 45, who died of gangrene of the lungs following removal of the tongue. (By Hamdi, *Deutsch. med. Woch.*, 1906, **32**: 1410.)

Fig. 6.—Right aortic arch with total suppression of left. The aorta is a large trunk 8 cm. in circumference, which gives off the left innominate from its anterior surface and curves upward and directly backward, descending on

the right of the vertebral column to the abdomen. Just beyond the origin of the right subclavian on its left wall is a tent-shaped diverticulum attached to a long ligamentum arteriosum which passes to it from the left branch of the pulmonary artery behind the trachea and oesophagus, thus enclosing these viscera in a vascular ring. Accidental finding in a woman aged 61 years, dying from intestinal obstruction. (Diagrammatic sketch by Prof. J. G. Adami from specimen No. 15.11[1] in the McGill Museum, Reported by M. E. Abbott, *Osler's Mod. Med.*, 1927, **4**: 791.)

Fig. 7.—Right aortic arch with persistent left aortic root supplying branches to both lungs in a case of pulmonary atresia. The large aorta 3.5 cm. in diameter rises above a defect in the interventricular septum and after giving off the left innominate and right branches arches down behind the right bronchus. Just opposite the left subclavian it gives off a flaring thin-walled tube, the dilated patent ductus, which communicates with a branch of the atresic pulmonary artery and empties into the hilum of the right lung. 2.5 cm. below this there rises from the left wall of the thoracic aorta a thick-walled left aortic root which passes up to the left, giving off two branches to the right and then to the left lung and apparently ending as a left subclavian artery. *a*, right aortic arch; *b*, patent ductus; *c*, varicose pulmonary end of *b*; left common carotid artery; *e*, anomalous left subclavian; *f*, trachea; *g*, pulmonary branch to right lung; *h*, oesophagus. From a man aged 29 with cyanosis, and clubbing, the result of the associated anomalies. (Case of Digby Wheeler, and M. E. Abbott, *Canad. Med. Assn. J.*, 1928, **19**: 297.)

Fig. 8.—Origin of right subclavian artery from descending arch of aorta. *a*, anterior; *b*, posterior view. The anomalous vessel originating from the posterior aspect of the aorta 5 mm. to the right of and below the left subclavian (*b*), ascended obliquely to the left crossing behind the oesophagus and trachea, which it pressed upon but did not constrict. An accidental finding in a woman aged 36, dying of pulmonary tuberculosis. (By Vera Dolgopol, *J. Tech. Meth.* 1934, **13**: 112.)

Fig. 9.—Absence of right pulmonary artery and replacement by anomalous branch from innominate and bleeding into right lung. Heart and lung of a well-developed somewhat cyanotic infant aged 6 days. The main pulmonary trunk continues directly into the descending aorta through the widely patent ductus and gives off, just before this, the right pulmonary artery to the lung of that side. The right pulmonary is replaced by a large vessel which passes from the innominate artery to the hilum of the right lung. This organ is cyanotic, cystic and microscopically shows extensive haemorrhage into the alveoli, due probably to the high systemic pressure acting upon the pulmonary capillaries in the congenital absence of the right pulmonary artery. The anomaly is explained as a too early involution of the right sixth arch and the substitution in the fourth embryonic week of an anomalous artery from the right fifth arch. *a*, pulmonary trunk; *b*, ascending aorta; *c*, left pulmonary artery; *d*, patent ductus arteriosus; *e*, aortic arch; *f*, innominate artery; *g*, anomalous right pulmonary artery from innominate to right lung. (Reported by G. Ambrus, *J. Tech. Meth.*, 1936, **5**: 103.)

PLATE VI. ANOMALIES OF THE AORTIC ARCH AND ITS BRANCHES

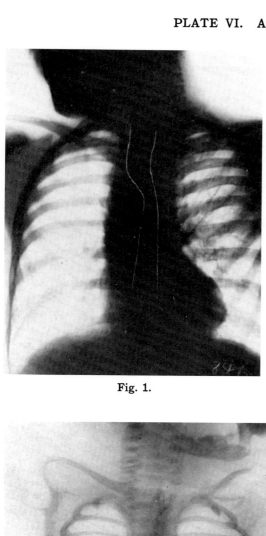

Fig. 1.

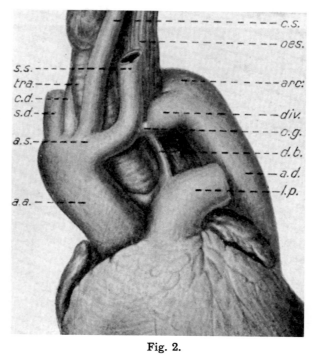

Fig. 2.

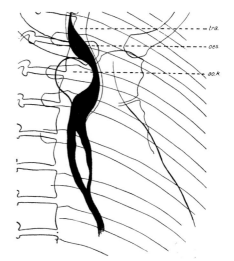

Fig. 3.

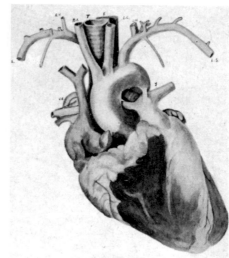
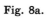

Fig. 8a.

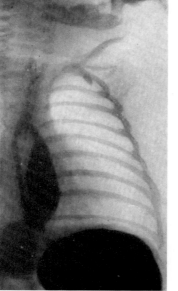

Fig. 4.

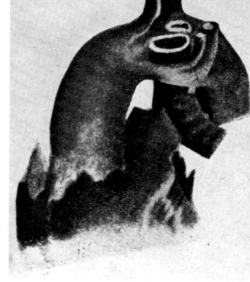
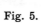

Fig. 5.

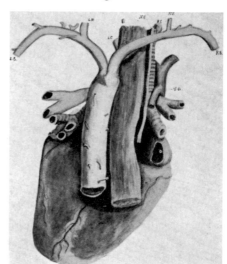

Fig. 8b.

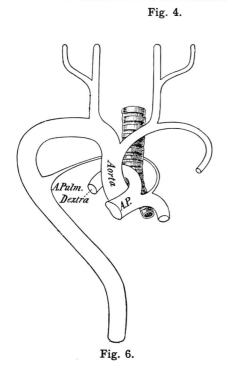

Fig. 6.

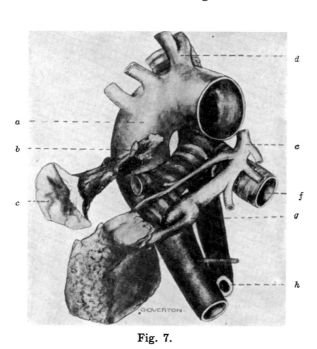

Fig. 7.

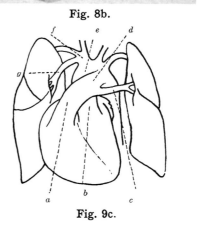

Fig. 9c.

PLATE VII

COARCTATION OF THE AORTA OF THE ADULT TYPE. HISTORIC CASES

CULLED FROM THE LITERATURE TO ILLUSTRATE THE PATHOLOGY OF THIS LESION

General Considerations. In this condition there is a more or less abrupt narrowing, constriction, or obliteration of the descending arch in the region of the insertion of the (usually obliterated) ductus arteriosus, with resultant formation of an extensive collateral circulation between the branches given off from the aorta *above* and those *below* the seat of coarctation. The aortic intercostal arteries play an important part in the development of these anastomotic channels and, by the continuous pulsation of their tortuous dilated channels against the adjacent compact bone, produce extensive *excavations in the borders of the ribs*, a conspicuous pathological change that was *first described and figured by Meckel in* 1827 (Fig. 3b) and which, when present, is plainly visible by the x-rays (Pl. VIII, Fig. 9). The ascending aorta is usually dilated and the aortic valve is frequently bicuspid. A dramatic termination by rupture of the aorta (Fig. 6), cerebral haemorrhage or other sudden lethal event (Fig. 5) is not uncommon; or life may be prolonged to an advanced age even in cases of extreme constriction, in the presence of a highly developed collateral circulation—as witness Reynaud's patient, a man who lived without apparent inconvenience to the age of 92 (Fig. 1). There is a curious predominance in the male sex (147 out of 200 cases analyzed, i.e., 70 per cent), and the subjects are usually highly developed individuals, of more than average intelligence and of great bodily vigor.

The extensive earlier literature was reviewed and illustrative cases published by J. T. King (*Arch. Int. Med.*, 1926, **38**: 69); W. F. Hamilton and M. E. Abbott (*Amer. Heart J.*, 1928, **3**: 381, 514); and L. M. Blackford (*Arch. Int. Med.*, 1928, **41**: 702). Rare instances of stricture of the aorta some distance below the ductus in the thoracic or abdominal aorta have been reported, by Schlesinger (*Wchnsch. f. d. ges. Heilk.*, 1835, p. 489); Hasler (*Leipzig Thesis*, 1911); Costa (*Arch. d. Pat. e. Clin. Med.*, 1929–30, **9**: 305) and W. H. Maycock of Montreal (in press). Attention is also drawn to the valuable recent contributions by H. Roesler (*Wien. Arch. f. inn. Med.*, 1928, **15**: 521) and William Evans (*Quart. J. Med.*, 1933, **16**: 205); and to the highly illuminating article by Sir Thomas Lewis (*Heart*, 1933, **16**: 205), in which complete blood vascular studies and electrocardiographic and x-ray tracings are presented for nine cases of coarctation, in eight of whom the diagnosis was made during life. See also the report of May G. Wilson (with diagnostic roentgenograms, *Amer. J. Dis. Child.*, 1932, **44**: 390); and that of W. E. Pierce (*J.A.M.A.*, 1934, **103**: 838, (mycotic aneurysm at seat of coarctation).

Fig. 1.—The collateral circulation in a case of extreme coarctation of the descending arch just below the ductus in a man dying at the age of 92. Note the anastomosis of the hugely dilated three upper aortic intercostals with the superior intercostal artery and the dilated and tortuous internal mammaries with the deep epigastrics. (From A. Reynaud, "Observation d'une oblitération presque complète de l'aorte, etc.," *J. hebd. de med.*, 1828, **1**: 161.)

Fig. 2.—Drawings from the injected cadaver showing details of the collateral circulation in a case of atresia of the descending arch two lines below the obliterated ductus in a man aged 21, a butcher by trade, who died suddenly from *rupture of a dissecting aneurysm* of the dilated ascending aorta.

a. Dissection of the arm and shoulder from this case showing the dilated and tortuous subscapular branch of the brachial artery emerging below the angle of the scapula to pierce the intercostal space posteriorly on its way to join the upper aortic intercostals.

b. The dilated epigastric arteries coursing down interiorly on either side of the sternum to anastomose with the internal mammaries. (From J. Jordan, "A case of obliteration of the aorta with disease of the valves," *North of Eng. M. and S. J.*, 1930, **1**: 101.)

Fig. 3.—**Meckel's case of extreme coarctation** of the descending arch admitting only a straw with enormous development of the collateral circulation in a Bernoise peasant, aged 29, who died six days after carrying a heavy bag of corn to market, *from rupture of the right auricle into the pericardium.*

a. Outline drawing of the aortic arch showing gradual narrowing of the isthmus with marked constriction just below the insertion of the ligamentum arteriosum and dilatation of the ascending aorta.

b. Dissection of the interior of the thoracic cavity to show the extraordinarily dilated and tortuous collaterals, especially the transverse cervicals and suprascapular branches of the subclavian artery and the anastomosis of the latter with the hugely dilated and tortuous intercostals and the excavations made in the ribs by these, as pointed out by this author. (From A. Meckel, "Verschliessung der Aorta am vierten Brustwirbel," *Arch. f. Anat. u. Phys.*, 1827, 345.)

Fig. 4.—A sudden constriction as though by a ligature just below the obliterated ductus, corresponding internally to a circular diaphragm 1 mm. thick with a central opening admitting a fine sound. The aorta expanded widely below the stricture, the ascending aorta, innominate and left subclavian also much dilated. Persistent left superior cava. In a farmer, age 27 years, dying of failing compensation. (From L. M. Bonnet, "Sur la lesion dite stenose congènitale de l'aorte dans la region de l'isthme," *Rev. de méd.*, Paris, 1903, **23**: 108.)

This article summarized all the important cases to date and presented a valuable review of the earlier literature.

Fig. 5.—Complete obliteration of the descending arch half an inch in length, beginning just below the insertion of the obliterated ductus with huge collateral circulation, in an Austrian officer, who had fought through the French Revolution and had suffered for the last year from dyspnoea, dysphagia and oedema of the extremities and died suddenly. (From A. Roemer, "Eine vollständige Verschliessung der Aorta bei einem 50-jährigen Manne," *Med. Jahrb. d. k. k. Oesterr. Staates*, 1839, **29**: 208.)

Fig. 6.—Extreme stenosis of the descending arch just below the insertion of the obliterated ductus with congenitally bicuspid aortic valve in a beautiful girl of 17, who had been apparently quite well except for occasional precordial distress and who became very ill with pain and loss of consciousness after rising suddenly in the night and walking across a cold room in bare feet to attend a sick relative, and died suddenly 8 hours later. Autopsy showed the ascending aorta greatly dilated and provided with only two cusps and presented on its left wall a jagged tear about 1 in. long beginning ½ in. behind the left coronary orifice and running obliquely upward, through which *rupture into the pericardium* had taken place. (From A. W. Otto, "Eine Zerreissung der Aorta, wegen stellenweiser grosser Verengerung derselben," in *Seltene Beobachtungen zur Anat. Phys. u. Path.*, 1824, p. 66.)

Fig. 7.—Extreme stenosis of the aorta at the level of the ductus which barely admitted a fine probe. The first aortic intercostals are seen dilated as are also the vessels of the arch. A beautifully depicted case. (From J. Cruveilhier, "Rétrécissement par froncement de l'aorte sans altération des parois," *Anat. path. du corps humain*, 1835–42, **43**, Fig. 3.)

PLATE VII. COARCTATION OF THE AORTA OF THE ADULT TYPE. HISTORIC CASES

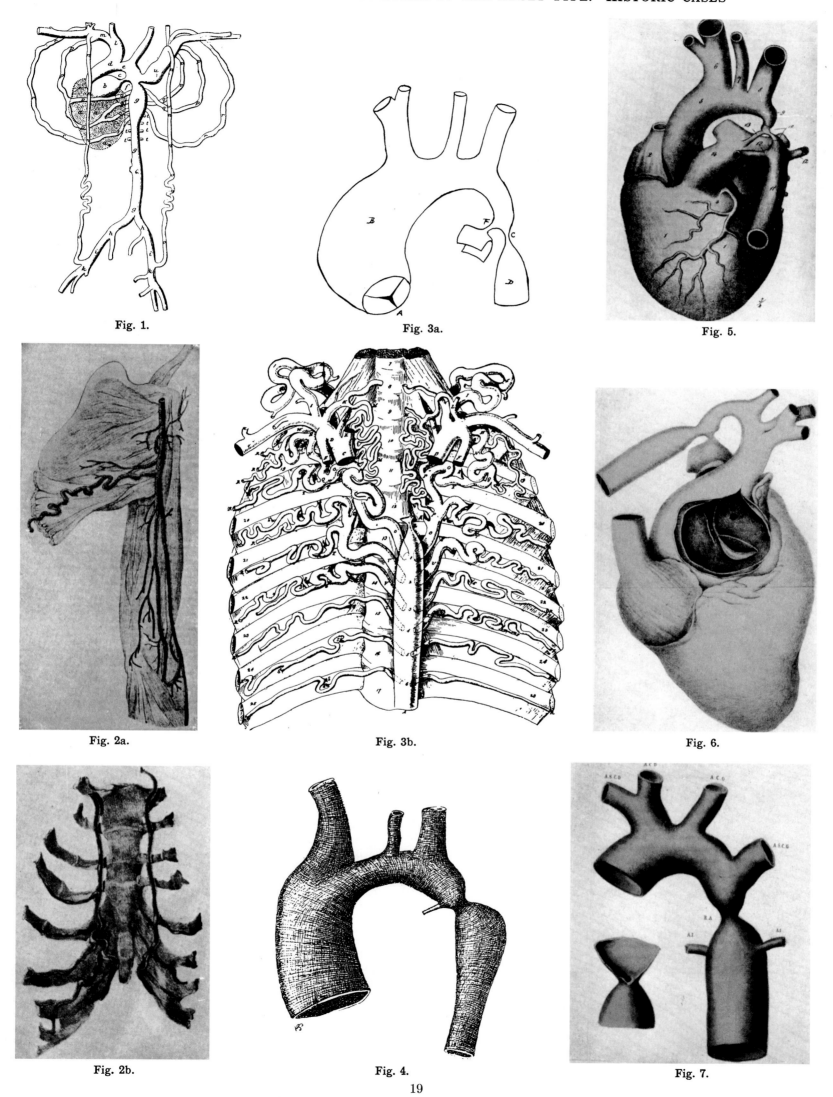

Fig. 1.

Fig. 3a.

Fig. 5.

Fig. 2a.

Fig. 3b.

Fig. 6.

Fig. 2b.

Fig. 4.

Fig. 7.

PLATE VIII

COARCTATION OF THE AORTA (*Continued*). PERSONAL CASES AND CLINICAL FEATURES

General Considerations. The interference with the main part of the circulation by the constriction in the descending arch and the consequent dilatation of the collaterals above the obstruction give rise to a series of vascular signs and of x-ray findings that are of pathognomonic value. Such are the hypertension that invariably exists in the upper part of the body along with reduction of *pressure* in the *lower* extremities, the *diminution* or absence of the femoral or popliteal pulse to the palpating finger and the relatively slow rise of the latter in the sphygmographic tracing (Figs. 7a and b); the disappearance over the upper part of the thorax and neck of *visible pulsations* in the tortuous and dilated collaterals, which often transmit also a fine thrill and systolic or postsystolic murmur; the *erosion of the ribs* (see Fig. 3), which is visible by x-rays in all cases in which it has occurred (Roesler's sign); and other roentgenological features, such as the peculiar contour of the left border of the cardiac shadow, the widened right base and the complete absence in the left oblique diameter of the descending arch (Fig. 6). Multiple capillary aneurysms seen in two carefully investigated cases were reported by Roesler as of diagnostic value (*Wien. Arch. f. inn. Med.*, 1928, **15**: 521).

Fig. 1.—Complete atresia of the descending arch with large collateral circulation, saccular aneurysm of ascending arch with impending rupture, congenitally bicuspid aortic valve and aortic insufficiency. Cerebral death.*

a. Anterior view, showing the enormously dilated and hypertrophied left ventricle laid open to reveal its interior, the sclerosed and incompetent bicuspid aortic valve, the dilatation of the ascending aorta, and the displacement of the great trunks to the extreme left of the elongated transverse arch.

a, the narrow aortic isthmus giving off an anomalous vessel; *b*, the area of complete obliteration at the level of *c*, the ligamentum arteriosum; *d*, interior of pulmonary artery; *e*, enlarged periarterial gland.

b. Posterior view of aortic arch and interior of dissective aneurysm. Just beyond the great trunks the aortic isthmus narrows rapidly to a ring of further constriction which coincides internally with a complete obliteration, the aorta above and below this point ending blindly in a shallow biconcave disc lined with shining healthy intima, indicating arrest of the fourth left arch at its junction with the sixth. The aorta below this area widens rapidly and presents the dilated orifices of the upper aortic intercostals.

From a boy of high intelligence, aged 14, who presented the characteristic clinical picture of coarctation with huge development of the collateral circulation, and died in coma setting in 12 hours before death. The brain was not examined, but cerebral haemorrhage was undoubtedly the cause. (Reported by W. F. Hamilton and M. E. Abbott, *Amer. Heart J.*, 1928, **3**: 381; 574. Drawings by H. Blackstock, Medical Art Department, McGill University.)

Fig. 2.—Coarctation of the aorta with double stricture of descending arch, bicuspid aortic valve, aortic, mitral and tricuspid stenosis and aortic and mitral insufficiency.* Sudden death.

A. Inner and outer views of the transverse and descending arch. Just beyond the left subclavian it has become abruptly narrowed (upper stricture) and then widens to undergo again at the level of the obliterated ductus a second very sharp kinking which corresponds internally to a thickened intimal ridge or shelf, enclosing a very narrow lumen. The aorta between these two points is ballooned out and twisted on itself. Below the second stricture it widens rapidly and attains after receiving the collateral supply through the dilated aortic intercostals a circumference of 56 mm.

B. Heart showing a marked simple hypertrophy of the left ventricle with dilatation and hypertrophy of both auricles, especially the right. The bicuspid aortic valve presents a low raphe behind the combined coronary segments and both segments are greatly thickened and manifestly incompetent.

From a primipara aged 34, who presented signs of cardiac insufficiency during her pregnancy and was successfully delivered by cesarian section in the eighth month of a viable baby, but died quietly in her sleep six nights later. (Report from the Pathological Service of the Royal Victoria Hospital, kindly supplied by W. H. Chase. Published by M. E. Abbott, *Libman Ann. Vol.*, 1932, **1**: 1. Drawing by H. Blackstock, Medical Art Department, McGill University.)

Fig. 3.—Roentgenograph in antero-posterior diameter of the heart and aortic arch from the case in Fig. 1, showing great broadening and convexity to right of the aortic shadow, and the characteristic contour of the left border with absence of aortic knob and kinking in the region of the aortic isthmus, also *erosion of the ribs*. (From *Amer. Heart J.*, 1928, **3**: 385, Fig. 1.)

Fig. 4.—The dilated and tortuous internal mammary arteries as they pass down to anastomose with the deep epigastrium in the upkeep of the collateral circulation. (*Ibid.*, p. 389, Fig. 4.)

Fig. 5.—Vascular signs. Markings in heavy charcoal on the back of a living case of coarctation, indicating the position of forcible pulsations in the dilated and tortuous branches of the dorsalis scapulae, supra- and subscapular arteries.

From a carpenter aged 58, with hypertension in the upper extremities, diminished femoral pulse and large collateral circulation, diagnosed during life from these features. (Republished by permission from the article by J. T. King, *Arch. Int. Med.*, 1926, **38**: 99.)

Fig. 6.—Roentgenograph in the left oblique diameter in Roesler's case of coarctation in a man of 45, who died suddenly in his sleep. The picture shows the ascending aorta dilated and passing backward toward the vertebral column at what appears to be a somewhat higher level than usual. In the retroaortic and retrocardiac space below it, the bifurcation of the trachea and one bronchus are clearly visible anteriorly, but behind these the area that is normally crossed by the descending arch is occupied by a clear space, the shadow of the descending arch being absent in this situation. (From H. Roesler, *Wien. Arch. f. inn. Med.*, 1928, **15**: 520, Fig. 3.)

Fig. 7.—Polygraphic tracings from the radial and femoral arteries and collaterals of the back, in Roesler's Case 2 of coarctation.

a. The femoral curve is much lower than in the radial and arises slowly and falls gradually, producing an elevation with an obtuse flattened top, and the rise begins a little later than that of the radial.

b. The curve in the collaterals is still shallower but the rise begins synchronously with that in the radial pulse. (From H. Roesler, *ibid.*, Fig. 5.)

Fig. 8.—Polygraphic tracings from the brachial and femoral arteries in a patient diagnosed clinically as coarctation. Note the difference in form, the slow up-stroke and low amplitude of the femoral as compared with the radial tracing. (From Laubry and Pezzi, *Traité des maladies congènitales du coeur*, 1921, p. 263, Fig. 94.)

Fig. 9.—Roentgenogram of thorax, showing marked erosion of the fourth to eighth ribs on both sides, in an unpublished case of coarctation, under the care of Douglas Wilkinson of Birmingham, England. The patient was a young man of 21, well built and powerful, a football and cricket player. Routine physical examination revealed a systolic pressure of 280 degrees with a diastolic so low that it could not be made out satisfactorily and no pulse palpable in the iliacs or abdominal aorta. Heart action was forcible but the organ was hardly enlarged. The diagnosis was made on the above characteristic findings. (From the copy kindly supplied by Dr. Wilkinson for this Atlas.)

Fig. 10.—Dr. Libman's case of mycotic aneurysm of the thoracic aorta just below the seat of coarctation with rupture into the left bronchus.

From a girl of 12, who died with symptoms of bacteraemia of one month's duration. Autopsy showed abundant streptococcus haemolyticus in the walls and thrombotic contents of the aneurysm, with subacute glomerulonephritis and embolism of femoral artery. (Reported by permission by M. E. Abbott, *Blumer's Bedside Diag.*, 1928, **3**: 376, Fig. 258. Drawing by A. Feinberg.)

Fig. 11.—Ruptured cerebral aneurysm thought to be congenital. This patient was an apparently healthy young man of 24, who fell on the street in an epileptiform convulsion and was brought into hospital in coma and died a few hours later. The base of the brain was enveloped in abundant haemorrhage, and dissection showed this small thin-walled sac at the second bifurcation of the anterior cerebral artery torn across on its free surface. Microscopic examination showed intimal proliferation and some medial degeneration. There was no coarctation but the case illustrates a not infrequent complication of this. (From C. P. Symonds, "Spontaneous subarachnoid haemorrhage," *Quart. J. Med.*, 1924–25, **18**: 118, Case 2.)

* Specimen in the Cardiac Anomaly Collection of McGill University.

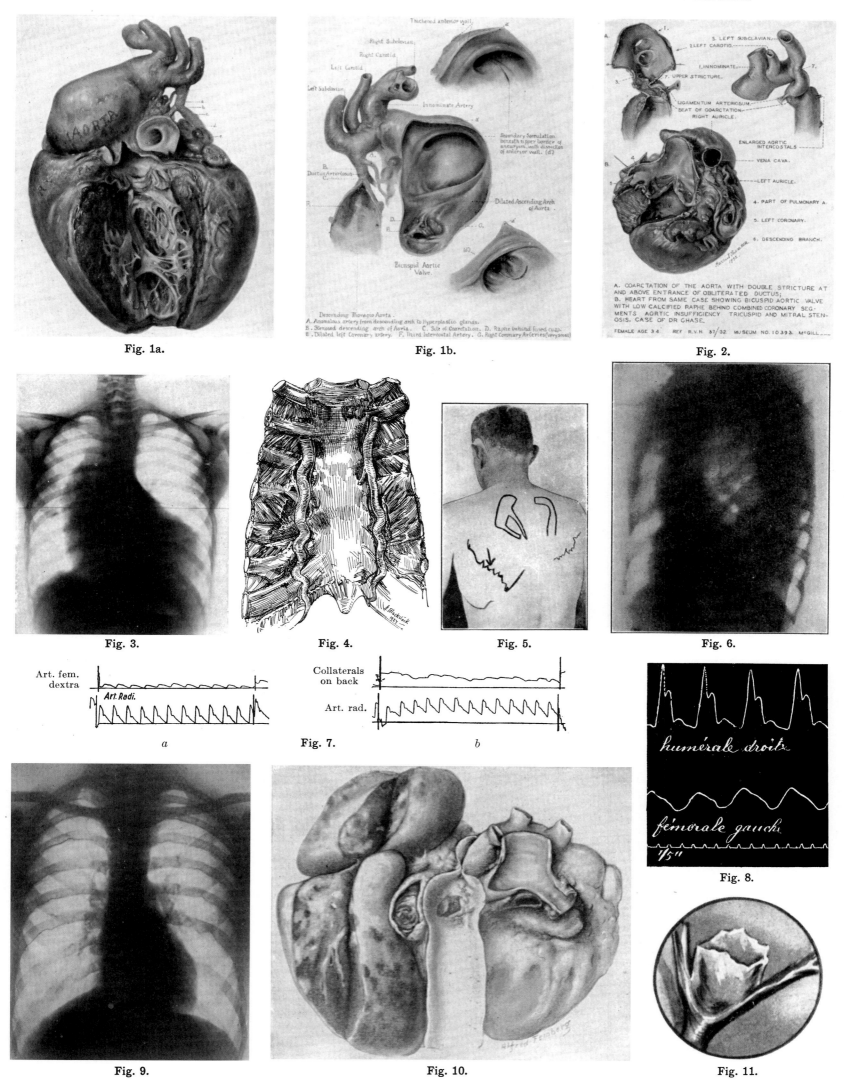

Fig. 1a.

Fig. 1b.

Fig. 2.

Fig. 3.

Fig. 4.

Fig. 5.

Fig. 6.

Fig. 7.

Fig. 8.

Fig. 9.

Fig. 10.

Fig. 11.

PLATE IX

A. BICUSPID AORTIC VALVE. B. SUPERNUMERARY AORTIC CUSPS

A. Congenitally bicuspid aortic valve is a relatively rare condition which does not of itself produce signs or symptoms. Nevertheless its presence is of serious clinical significance on account of the fact that it almost invariably undergoes sclerotic changes and becomes the seat of a subacute bacterial endocarditis usually with lethal results (Fig. 8); or the ascending aorta immediately above the valve may undergo dilatation with dissection of its coats and secondary rupture into the pericardium (Figs. 6, 9, 10). It is important therefore to differentiate between a congenital union and a postnatal inflammatory fusion. The macroscopic features distinctive of a congenital origin were first pointed out by Sir William Osler in 1880 and again in 1886 in a careful morphological and statistical study of 16 personal cases; the microscopic criteria however, which alone can furnish positive evidences in doubtful cases, were first established by Sir T. Lewis and R. T. Grant (1923) in their brilliant histological investigation of the architecture of (a) the normal and (b) the conjoint segments. In it they show that the normal reversal of the annulus fibrosus with the elastica of the aortic media which takes place at this area is absent in the abortive commissure, the annulus remaining submerged beneath the elastica which may pass over superficially in an unbroken layer, or undergoes a confused whorling. Similar observations on the structure of the commissure were recorded by Gross and Kugel (*Amer. J. Path.*, 1931, **7**: 445) and recently by Bishop and Trubek (Fig. 5).

Fig. 1.—**Diagram by Lewis and Grant of the structures supporting the normal aortic valve.** Serial reconstruction made from vertical sections taken through the entire breadth of the aortic lumen. The stippling represents the aortic media, the vertical lines the annulus fibrosus, *A.F.*; the heavy black line, *F.V.*, indicates the fibrous layer of the valves; *D.E.* the deep and *S.E.* the superficial endings of the elastica of the media; *M.S.*, membranous septum; *M.V.*, mitral valve; *R.A.*, *P.*, and *L.A.*, the right anterior, posterior, and left anterior cusps; *A*, *B*, and *C*, the commissures formed at the junction of the right and left anterior, right anterior and posterior, and at junction of posterior and left anterior cusps; *R.C.* and *L.C.*, the two coronary arteries. Note that here the normal reversal has occurred, the annulus emerging from below and passing superficially to the deep elastica over the top of each commissure.

Fig. 2.—**Diagram of the structures supporting a congenitally bicuspid aortic valve with no trace of raphe.** Serial reconstruction by these authors from a specimen in the Museum of University College. Lettering as in Fig. 1. Note that at the site of the abortive commissure the annulus fibrosus lies deep to the elastica, the latter sweeping superficially over the floor of the sinus behind the composite cusp and curving over the slight elevation produced by the (displaced) membranous septum. (From article by T. Lewis and R. T. Grant, *Heart*, 1923, **10**: 23, 35, Figs. 1 and 2.)

Fig. 3.—**Peacock's case of congenital bicuspid aortic valve with union of right anterior and posterior cusps (commissure B) and partial fusion of anterior segments.** The aortic arch laid open to show the deformed aortic valve which is irregularly thickened and the sinus behind the conjoint cusp unequally divided by a prominent raphe. The ascending aorta is dilated and the descending arch is narrowed in the isthmus region but undergoes a bulbous dilatation after entrance of the patent ductus. Female infant, aged 10 weeks. (Specimen in the Museum of University College, described and figured by Thomas B. Peacock in his *Malformations of the Human Heart*, 2d ed., 1866, p. 152, Pl. viii, Fig. 1. Congenital origin confirmed by Lewis and Grant Fig. 4 below.)

Fig. 4.—**Microphotograph of serial section taken by Lewis and Grant through the abortive commissure in Peacock's case of bicuspid aortic valve demonstrating its congenital origin.** The main ridge (*r*) is seen rising above a central space which is the normal projection upward of the ventricular cavity below the commissure and is lined by endocardium containing a strong layer of elastic tissue (*V.e.*, ventricular elastica). Externally to this the fibrous layer of the valve is continuous with the annulus fibrosus (*an.f.*), and the whole ridge is covered on its aortic surface with a thin layer of elastic tissue (*S.e.*) which is continuous on either side with the aortic media, and is itself in part covered superficially by a layer of foetal connective tissue representing a much thickened subendothelial layer (*V.s.*). "*These observations stamp the deformity as a congenital malformation, for they clearly show that the two cusps have been laid down in one sheet without subdivision.*" (From the article by Lewis and Grant, *ibid.*, pp. 32–33, Fig. 8.)

Fig. 5a.—**Microphotograph of a serial transverse section through the raphe of a bicuspid aortic valve due to inflammatory fusion, showing normal commissural relationships.** Note that the connective tissue of the annulus passes superficially to the aortic media to form the apex of the commissure, while the deep layers of the elastica pass uninterrupted below the annulus, the normal reversal existing. From a man aged 45 with advanced aortic stenosis with calcification of cusps, dying from congestive failure.

Fig. 5b.—**Transverse serial section through raphe of a congenitally bicuspid aortic valve showing lack of normal reversal.** A layer of connective tissue (the abortive annulus) appears below the whorled elastic fibers of the media which lie superficially. Male, aged 26. Coronary cusps fused, raphe almost obliterated. Accidental finding in death from bullet wound. (From L. F. Bishop and M. Trubek, *J. Tech. Meth.*, 1936, **15**: 123, Fig. V, and 119, Fig. III *C*.)

Fig. 6.—**Bicuspid aortic valve with fusion of right anterior and posterior segments (commissure B) and huge saccular aneurysm of right anterior sinus of Valsalva eroding sternum and rupturing externally.** Atheroma and dilatation of ascending aorta, aortic insufficiency.* (Reported by M. E. Abbott, *Libman Ann. Vol.*, 1932, **1**: 23.)

Fig. 7.—**Four of Osler's 16 cases of bicuspid aortic valve believed to be congenital, showing a raphe of varying height behind the conjoint segment and aortic incompetency. a. Fusion of coronary segments with low almost obliterated raphe.** The conjoint segment is defective at its right posterior end from ulcerative endocarditis and is here anchored to the aortic wall by a tendinous cord. From a blacksmith, aged 26, dying from cardiac dropsy.

b. Fusion of coronary cusps with high raphe, the conjoint shorter than the single segment. Chronic infective endocarditis with calcification of vegetations and multiple valvular aneurysms. From a man aged 45, dying with symptoms of severe aortic valvular disease.*

c. Fusion of coronary cusps with low raphe, the fused shorter than the single segment. Ulcerative endocarditis with perforation of single segment. From a young man, aged 20, who presented symptoms of acute endocarditis but died suddenly of ruptured cerebral aneurysm (? congenital).*

d. Fusion of anterior segments with low raphe and V-shaped deficiency in the conjoint curtain. The single cusp longer than the conjoint segment. From a man aged 42, dying of cardiac dropsy after 5 months' illness. (Reported by William Osler with four other cases in the *Montreal General Hosp. Repts. Clin. and Path.*, 1880, **1**: 233, Pl. IX. Author's cases I, V, II, and IV respectively. Republished by him with eight additional cases, *Tr. Amer. Assn. Phys.*, 1886, **1**: 185.)

Fig. 8.—**Congenitally bicuspid aortic valve with fusion of coronary cusps and almost obliterated raphe, insufficiency of segments, and infective endocarditis and mycotic aneurysm of circumflex branch of left coronary artery rupturing into wall of left auricle with extensive myocardial infarction of left ventricle.*** Associated subaortal septal defect, hypoplasia and coarctation of aorta. From a tall spare man, aged 34, who presented a musical systolic murmur (generated at the defect) but was in good health until the last year. Symptoms of bacterial endocarditis two months and repeated anginal attacks of increasing severity, in one of which he died. Blood culture was negative, but abundant streptococci in the vegetations and in wall of aneurysm. (From a case in the service of D. S. Lewis. Reported by M. E. Abbott and W. H. Chase, *J. Tech. Meth.*, 1929, **12**: 171.)

Fig. 9.—**Bicuspid aortic valve with calcified raphe behind fused (coronary) cusps and great elongation of single segment, dilatation and dissecting aneuryms of ascending aorta rupturing into pericardium.** The aortic valve is calcified and insufficient and the heart in a state of marked eccentric hypertrophy. The right coronary orifice is displaced high above the aortic ring.* (Reported by M. E. Abbott, *Libman Ann. Vol., ibid.*, Case 2, p. 21, Fig. VI.)

B. Supernumerary Aortic Cusps

Fig. 10.—**Fourth aortic cusp of irregular triangular shape interposed between the two coronary segments and united with the left of these by a low raphe.** Saccular aneurysm of the sinus of Valsalva behind this combined segment with dissection of wall and impending rupture. Syphilitic mesaortitis with aortic sclerosis and insufficiency.* (Reported by M. E. Abbott, *ibid.*, Case 4, p. 29, Fig. IX.)

Fig. 11.—**Anomalous aortic valve. Fourth semilunar cusp fused with the left anterior one, the sinus behind these being incompletely divided by a high raphe.** The right anterior and posterior cusps show multiple fenestrations. No other anomalies or disease of the endocardium. From a man aged 21 who died of miliary tuberculosis. (Unpublished case of L. F. Bishop, Jr.)

* Specimen in the Cardiac Anomaly Collection of McGill University.

PLATE IX. A. BICUSPID AORTIC VALVE. B. SUPERNUMERARY AORTIC CUSPS

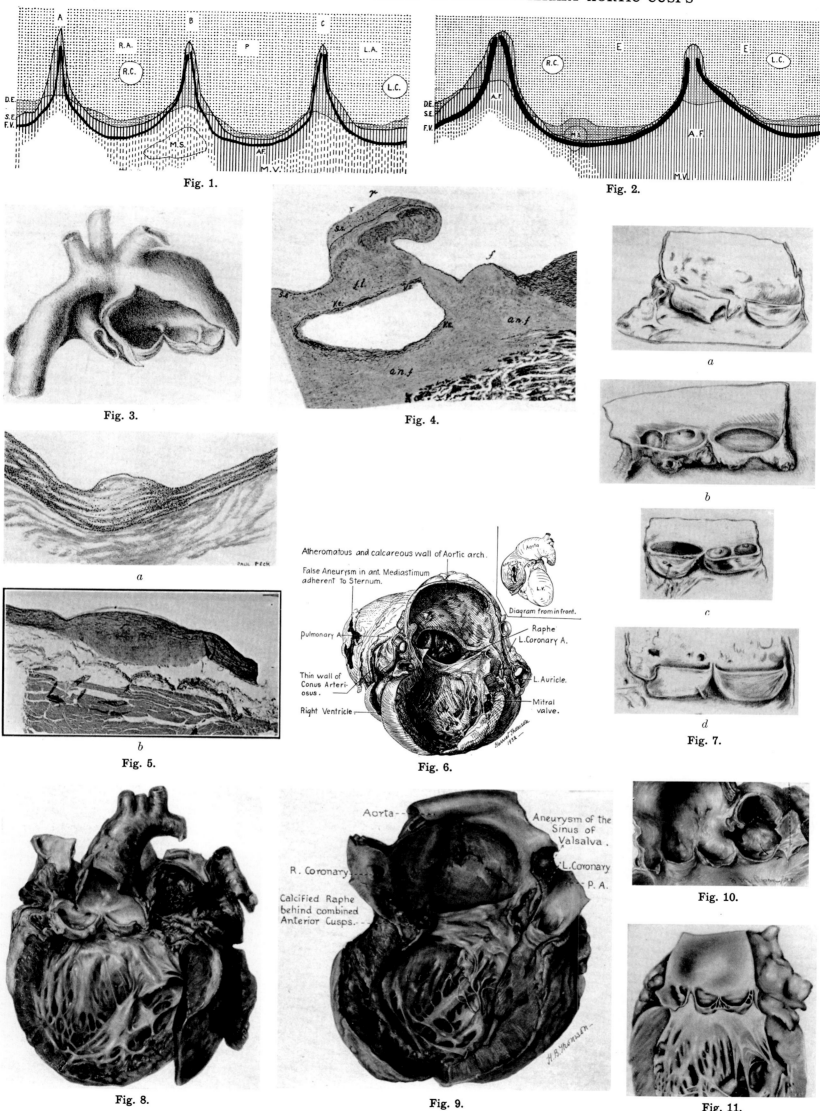

Fig. 1.

Fig. 2.

Fig. 3.

Fig. 4.

Fig. 5.

a

b

Fig. 6.

Atheromatous and calcareous wall of Aortic arch.

False Aneurysm in ant. Mediastimum adherent To Sternum.

Diagram from in front.

Pulmonary A.

Raphe

L.Coronary A.

Thin wall of Conus Arteriosus.

L. Auricle.

Right Ventricle

Mitral valve.

a

b

c

d

Fig. 7.

Fig. 8.

Aorta

Aneurysm of the Sinus of Valsalva.

R. Coronary

L.Coronary

P. A.

Calcified Raphe behind combined Anterior Cusps.

Fig. 9.

Fig. 10.

Fig. 11.

23

PLATE X

OTHER ANOMALIES OF THE ENDOCARDIUM

In contrast to the similar lesion at the aortic orifice, a *bicuspid pulmonary valve* is rare as an isolated anomaly but is relatively common in association with other defects, being a practically constant feature of the developmental type of pulmonary stenosis in the combination known as the "tetralogy of Fallot" (see Pl. IV and XIV). *Supernumerary pulmonary cusps*, on the other hand, four or even five in number, occur more frequently here than at the aortic orifice, but are not usually the seat of inflammatory changes so are not of much clinical import. Of the conditions figured opposite, *subaortic stenosis* (Fig. 1) does not in itself interfere with cardiac function but is nevertheless of serious significance on account of the fact that it is liable to become the seat of a subacute infective process as illustrated in the classic cases of Goldenweizer and Wiglesworth (in press). It can usually be readily differentiated from stenosis at the aortic orifice proper by the absence of any systemic evidence of aortic obstruction in the presence of distinctive physical signs at this area. *Aberrant chordae tendineae* (Fig. 2) are likewise of interest from the diagnostic standpoint on account of the confusing signs they are liable to produce but are unimportant otherwise. *Double mitral orifice*, a rare condition usually occurring with cleavage of the anterior mitral segment (Fig. 4), is apparently always latent, an accidental finding at autopsy. The same applies to *anomalous network* in the auricles (Fig. 3), although this has sometimes led to a lethal termination through becoming the seat of origin of embolism from thrombi lodged in their meshes. *Congenital tricuspid insufficiency*, on the other hand, is an extremely serious condition terminating in early infancy with generalized cyanosis. This properly belongs with the cyanotic group (III). The two chief anatomical types recognized are shown in Figs. 5a, b, c, and 6. *Congenital aortic and mitral stenosis of inflammatory origin* are rare left-sided lesions not shown in this Atlas.

Important additional references on the conditions figured opposite are the following: On subaortic stenosis: Thursfield and Scott, *Brit. J. Child. Dis.*, 1913, **10**: 104; Goldenweizer, *Med. Oborz. Mosk.*, 1912, **87**: 319; C. Sternberg, *Verh. d. deutsch. path. Gesell.*, 1930, **25**: 238. Aberrant chordae in ventricles: H. Huchard, *Rev. de méd.*, 1895, **13**, 113; Goforth, *J.A.M.A.*, 1926, **86**: 1612; Costa, *Clin. Med. Ital.*, 1930, **56**: 572. Anomalous network in right atrium: Chiari, *Zieg. Beitr.*, 1897, **22**: 1; W. W. Yater, *Arch. Path.*, 1929, **7**: 418; Helwig, *Amer. J. Path.*, 1932, **8**: 73.

Fig. 1.—Subaortic stenosis. In the rare and interesting condition here shown, the aortic ostium was not narrowed and its valves were completely competent, but a short distance below these a thick fibrous ridge, 2 cm. wide by 1.5 cm. high, projected into the cavity of the ventricle, traversing the base of the anterior mitral segment and forming a complete ring lining its interior. The left ventricle was hypertrophied, but the heart was otherwise normal. Young man aged 19 in good health since childhood. Admitted in second week of typhoid fever and died some months later of purulent pleurisy. Physical examination showed a systolic thrill in the third right interspace and a very long loud humming systolic murmur heard at all ostia but maximum over the upper sternum. Under observation in hospital the systolic vibration over the aortic area and great vessels became stronger and a short diastolic murmur developed at the apex. Coarctation was erroneously diagnosed. (Reported by J. H. Lindman, *Deutsch. Arch. f. klin. Med.*, 1880, **25**: 510, Pl. VI.)

Fig. 2.—Aberrant chordae tendineae in left ventricle producing a loud musical murmur audible 15 feet away from the patient. A cor bovinum of aortic insufficiency laid open to show the interior of the right ventricle, and an anomalous chorda, which, arising from one of the papillary muscles of the mitral valve, was attached high up on the ventricular surface of its aortic segment half an inch below the aortic cusp. Two other fine tendinous cords traversed the ventricle and joined the first at right angles, while a second passed to be attached to the ventricular wall close to the point of insertion of the first. From a laborer aged 40 years, who presented, in addition to the classic signs of aortic incompetency, a prolonged diastolic thrill over the third and fourth left interspaces, and a loud musical diastolic murmur maximum at the same area but plainly heard over the whole thorax and 15 to 24 feet from the chest wall. These signs diminished with the onset of congestive failure a few weeks before death. (Reported by W. F. Hamilton, *Montreal Med. J.*, July, 1899.)

Fig. 3.—Anomalous chordae ("network of Chiari") in right auricle. A system of fine tendinous threads attached to the lower border of the auricular septum, to the apex and body of the auricular surface of the tricuspid segment and to the right wall of the auricle just below the Eustachian valve. Probably vestigial remains of the valvula venosa dextra. (From F. C. Helwig, *Amer. J. Path.*, 1932, **8**: 73.)

Fig. 4.—Double mitral orifice. An enlarged heart laid open to show the auricular surface of the mitral valve. Its anterior segment is occupied about its middle by a perfectly formed secondary mitral orifice, formed by an ovoid cleft 2 cm. long, supplied with two delicate cusps which were attached by short but perfectly formed chordae to a group of papillary muscles situated high up on the anterior wall of the ventricle. The whole is an exact replica of the larger "primary" mitral orifice, and the two evidently functioned together. The segments of the latter valve are attached to a powerful group of papillary muscles springing from the left wall of the ventricle. An accidental finding in an old man aged 71, who died after amputation of the thigh for gangrene of the leg. *The renal artery and vein were double on both sides*, a suggestive combination. (From J. Cohn, *Über doppelte Atrio-ventricular-ostium*, Königsberg, 1896, p. 19, Pl. I.)

Fig. 5.—Congenital tricuspid insufficiency due to incomplete differentiation of septal cusps. *

a. Electrocardiogram from this case. Tracing shows a regular sinus rhythm with rate of 100. Right-axis deviation is marked. P_1 and P_2 of good amplitude, P_3 is frequently inverted. R_2 is low. A deep Q_3 is present. The R-T segment is slightly elevated in leads I and II. T_1 and T_2 are upright. *Impression:* Increased right auricular activity and right ventricular strain. (Reading by G. Nicolson.)

b. The heart laid open to show interior of the hugely dilated right chambers and the anomalous tricuspid valve. The marginal and infundibular segments are well developed and are attached by delicate chordae to well-formed papillary muscles, but the septal cusp is incorporated on its ventricular surface with the underlying myocardium without the intervention of these structures, and it carries on its auricular surface a mass of irregularly formed papillary endocardial outgrowths of gelatinous appearance arranged in rows along its free border and extending along the other cusps, as well as on the free borders of the pulmonary segments. The foramen ovale and ductus arteriosus are widely patent and the inferior cava has a triple orifice.

c. X-ray of this heart in the antero-posterior diameter, showing enormous enlargement of the cardiac shadow, which extends to the axillary borders and above to the second rib.

From a cyanotic male infant aged 7 days, who presented a rough presystolic thrill with accompanying presystolic and long rough systolic murmurs heard with maximum intensity over the center of the precordium a little to the left of the midsternal line. At autopsy the heart lay transversely against the diaphragm and completely filled the anterior aspect of the thorax, the hugely dilated right auricle and ventricle lying to the right and left of the auriculo-ventricular sulcus which ran obliquely downward in the median line of the body. The tricuspid orifice measured 7.5 cm., the pulmonary 2 cm. in circumference. Microscopic examination of the endocardial nodules on the tricuspid and pulmonary cusps showed these covered with a single layer of endothelium and to consist of an abundant fibrillary matrix continuous with the endocardium and showing no sign of inflammation or hyperplasia. (From an unpublished case under care of Graham Ross in the Royal Victoria Hospital, Montreal, from the autopsy service of Prof. Horst Oertel. Drawing by P. Larivière, Medical Art Department, McGill University.)

Fig. 6.—Ebstein type of congenital tricuspid insufficiency. A membranous sheet containing multiple large fenestrations is stretched across the orifice and displaced below the ring posteriorly, so that a part of the right ventricle lies in the cavity of the auricle, resulting in great dilatation of both chambers. (Case of J. Bassen of Yale. Reported by M. E. Abbott, *Blumer's Bedside Diag.*, 1928, **3**: 482.)

* Specimen in the Cardiac Anomaly Collection of McGill University.

PLATE X.   OTHER ANOMALIES OF THE ENDOCARDIUM

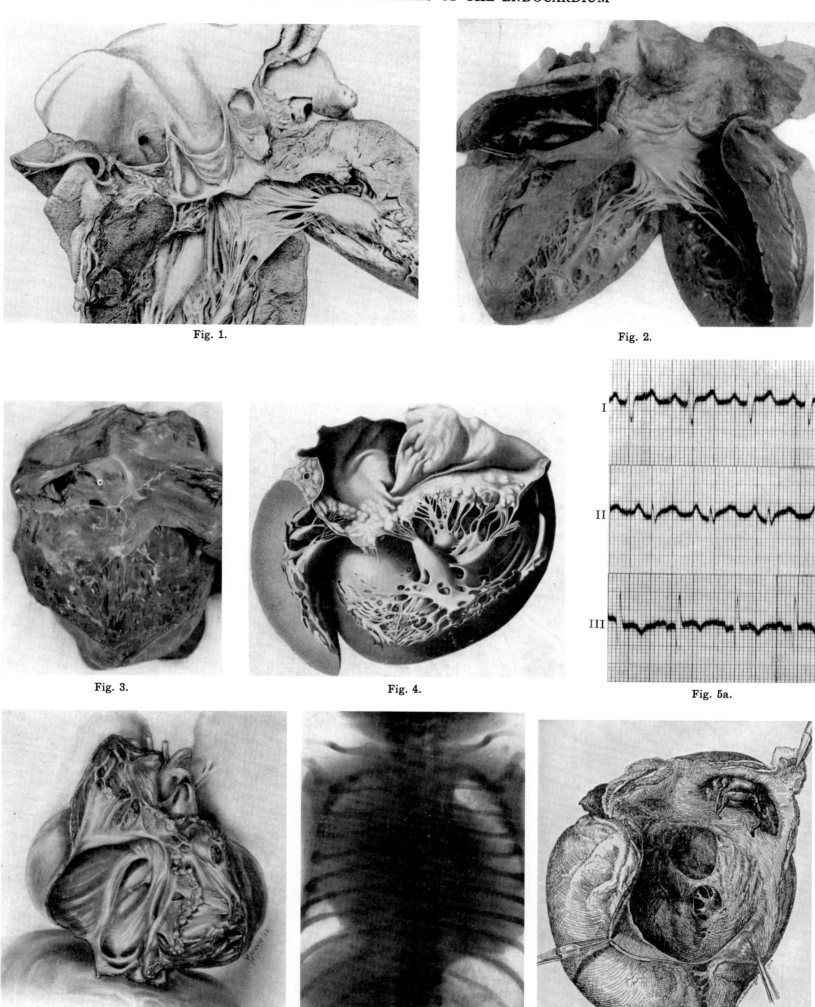

Fig. 1.

Fig. 2.

Fig. 3.

Fig. 4.

Fig. 5a.

Fig. 5b.

Fig. 5c.

Fig. 6.

PLATE XI

A. HYPERTROPHY OF THE HEART IN INFANTS. B. CONGENITAL RHABDOMYOMA

A. Hypertrophy of the Heart in Infants. The term "congenital idiopathic hypertrophy" has long been applied to a now well-recognized condition occurring in infancy and early childhood, characterized by great cardiac enlargement in the absence of any sign of myocardial disease or other intra- or extracardiac etiological factor, a pure or primary hypertrophy of the muscle fibers alone existing. This concept of the pathology of this condition has been gradually changing as a result of investigations into the history of the recorded cases and the more careful histological examination of the myocardium in those recently presented. Thus Stoloff, in 1928 in a statistical survey of the 34 cases in the literature at that date, eliminated all but 17 of these from the "idiopathic" class as presenting a definite etiology, and Kugel and Stoloff in 1933 got only 15 apparently primary hypertrophies from 52 cases analyzed. This number must undoubtedly be further reduced in the light of Putschar's and Pompe's recognition in 1933 of the cardiac type of glycogen-storage disease as a cause of congenital cardiomegaly; and also of the findings recorded in Kugel and Stoloff's recent monograph of definite inflammatory changes in the hearts of seven cases of massive cardiac enlargement occurring in children varying from 3 months to 6½ years in age. The latter authors express their belief that with our increasing knowledge of the causes of cardiac hypertrophy in children and with the help of a systematic microscopic investigation of the myocardium, in every case brought to autopsy, the old concept of the "idiopathic" nature of this lesion will eventually completely disappear. Congenital hypertrophy of the heart, presumably present at or before birth as in Simmonds' and Oberndorffer's early cases remains, however, a definite clinical entity, characterized by great cardiac enlargement, pallor and lassitude, the sudden onset of dyspnoea and cyanosis and a tendency to sudden dramatic exitus. The cases figured opposite are examples of some of the different pathological conditions that may underlie these phenomena. That shown in Fig. 1 (cardiomegaly glycogenica) was published by Paul White in 1931, two years before Putschar's article appeared.

B. Congenital rhabdomyoma (Fig. 2) is shown here in proximity to the latter case as featuring the suggestion brought forward by some authors that a similar perverted or delayed glycogen metabolism might be at work in both conditions.

In addition to the references cited below see the following: A. So-called primary congenital hypertrophy: Simmonds, *Münch. med. Woch.*, 1899, **46**: 108; Oberndorffer, *Monatschr. f. Kindheilk.*, 1914, **13**: 357; M. Steiner and M. Bogin, *Amer. J. Dis. Child.*, 1930, **39**: 1255; E. G. Stoloff, *Amer. J. Dis. Child.*, 1928, **36**: 1204; M. Kugel and E. G. Stoloff, *Amer. J. Dis. Child.*, 1933, **45**: 229. Cardiomegaly glycogenica: W. Putschar, *Beit. z. path. Anat. Zieg.*, 1932–33, **90**: 223; J. C. Pompe, *Ann. d'anat. path.*, 1933, **10**: 23; E. M. Humphreys and K. Kato, *Amer. J. Path.*, 1934, **10**: 589; A. B. Ellis, *Proc. Roy. Soc. Med. Sect. Dis. Child.*, 1934, **34**: 282, 1330. Cardiac hypertrophy in infancy in coarctation of aorta: H. D. Levine, *Amer. J. Dis. Child.*, 1934, **48**: 1072. Hypertension in a boy of 2 years; H. B. Taussig and D. Remsen, *Bull. Johns Hopkins Hosp.*, 1935, **57**: 183. B. Congenital rhabdomyoma: L. Berger and A. Vallée, *Ann. d'anat. path.*, 1930, **7**: 797; S. Farber, *Amer. J. Path.*, 1930, **7**: 105; W. M. Yater, *Arch. Int. Med.*, 1931.

Fig. 1.—Congenital so-called idiopathic hypertrophy, proved by microscopic investigation to be the seat of von Gierke's glycogen storage (cardiomegaly glycogenica). The liver, which was also enlarged, showed diffuse vacuolization of its cells.

a. Roentgenograph from this case showing great enlargement of the cardiac shadow, which fills the left chest merging with the shadow of pneumonic consolidation of the left lung.

b. The heart itself, showing great increase in size especially in its left chambers and a rounded globular contour. At autopsy it occupied one full third of the thorax and weighed 175 gm. (normal 34 gm.). Microscopic examination by Tracy Mallory showed the muscle cells twice as large as normal at this age, with large vacuoles surrounding the nucleus in each muscle cell, which did not react to fat stains but showed carmine-stained granules when treated later with Best reagents (see Humphrey and Kato, *Amer. J. Path.*, 1934, **10**: 599).

From a girl aged 7 months with an interesting familial history of congenital heart disease, who from the sixth month had had spells of quick breathing accompanied by cyanosis, and became markedly cyanotic 2 days before death, with high temperature and signs of lobar pneumonia. There was marked precordial prominence, and the electrocardiogram (the only one reported on in glycogenic cardiomegaly) showed sinoauricular tachycardia, rate 140, and normal axis deviation. (Reported by Sprague, Bland and White, *Amer. J. Dis. Child.*, 1931, **41**: 877. Fig. *b* reproduced from *Heart Disease* by Paul White, by permission of The Macmillan Company, New York.)

Fig. 2.—Congenital rhabdomyoma of the heart with multiple nodules in the myocardium of the right ventricle. From an infant aged 9 months which died in convulsions. At autopsy the tumors showed the characteristic histological structure, and there was tuberous sclerosis of the brain and kidneys. (Unpublished case in the service of K. Terplan of Buffalo. Specimen No. 14.142⁴ in the Cardiac Anomaly Collection of McGill University.)

Fig. 3.—Congenital hypertrophy of the heart in anomalous origin of the left coronary artery.

a. Electrocardiogram from this case showing low voltage and normal axis deviation with a late and deep inversion of the *T* waves of the coronary type, especially well seen in leads I and II. The latter feature yields definite diagnostic evidence in this combination of the anomalous origin of the left coronary, and the tracing is of great interest in that connection.

b. The heart laid open to show the cavity of the right ventricle. The orifice of the anomalous coronary is seen above the left pulmonary cusp. The curious arterio-venous dilatation shown in Pl. IV, Fig. 3 was in process of development, but is not visible in the picture.

c. Seven-foot x-ray film of the chest, showing the diffuse cardiac enlargement, most marked in the region of the left ventricle.

From a female child aged 3 months, well until 2 weeks before death, when paroxysmal attacks with difficult respiration, transient loss of consciousness and signs of severe shock set in. Death of respiratory failure some hours after one of these attacks. No cyanosis except on prolonged crying. The heart weighed 91 gm., left ventricle 11 mm. thick, left coronary from pulmonary artery, all branches dilated. Microscopic examination showed increase in number of muscle fibers, large vascular spaces with intervening fibrosis with myofibrillary degeneration at deeper levels and some vacuolization of individual cells. (Republished by permission from E. F. Bland, Paul D. White, and Jos. Garland, *Amer. Heart J.*, 1933, **8**: 787, Figs. 1, 2 and 4.)

Fig. 4.—Dilatation and hypertrophy of the heart with myocardial degeneration and fibrosis, in an infant aged 8 months.

a. The x-ray of this case shows a greatly enlarged cardiac shadow which reached to the axillary border on the left and the midclavicular line on the right. Shadow at the base also widened especially on left.

b. Anterior view of the enlarged heart. At autopsy it weighed 90 gm. (normal 32 gm.) and was distinctly dilated as well as hypertrophied in all its chambers with all valves normal.

c. Microphotograph of the myocardium showing focal areas of myocardial degeneration and a few lymphocytes around fibrous areas in the myocardium. Some of the muscle fibers showed atrophy and degeneration with replacement fibrosis. There were no areas of suppurative infiltration. A few muscle cells showed vacuoles giving a glycogen reaction.

d. Electrocardiogram showing sinus tachycardia rate about 150 beats per minute. *QRS* of low amplitude in lead I. *T* waves of low amplitude. (An unpublished case in the service of Maurice Kugel from the same series reported, *Amer. J. Dis. Child.*, 1930, **39**: 1255, and kindly supplied by him for publication in this Atlas.)

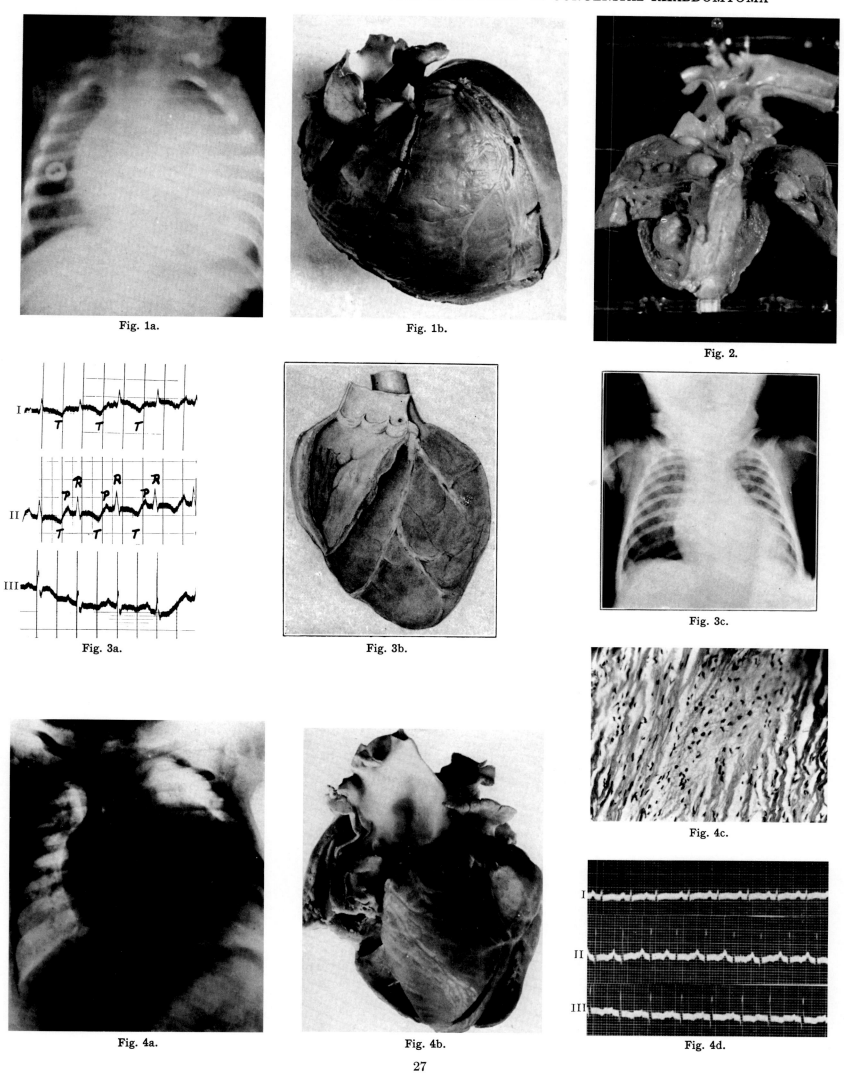

Fig. 1a.

Fig. 1b.

Fig. 2.

Fig. 3a.

Fig. 3b.

Fig. 3c.

Fig. 4c.

Fig. 4a.

Fig. 4b.

Fig. 4d.

27

PLATE XII

ANOMALIES OF THE CORONARY SINUS

The three remarkable cases figured opposite require a word of elucidation from the standpoint of development. The coronary sinus is derived from the transverse portion and left horn of the sinus venosus, which receives the left superior vena cava of later foetal life, and its proximal part persists in the normal human heart while the distal portion of the left superior vena cava undergoes involution but can still be traced in the tiny vestigial oblique vein of Marshall. Persistence of this entire trunk may occur as shown in Fig. 3. Further, the pulmonary veins originate as a single trunk in the center of the sinus venosus, but subsequently, on the shifting of this cavity to the right of the embryonic heart, come to lie in the posterior wall of the primitive auricle just to the *left* of the valvula venosa sinistra; and an arrest at this point, so that the common pulmonary vein remained in connection with the sinus venosus, would result in the very rare anomaly shown in Fig. 1. Lastly, Bela Halpert's case, shown in Fig. 2, is an exquisite example, unique in the literature, of a true congenital arterio-venous aneurysm of the coronary circulation, the result of an anomalous anastomosis in the primitive vascular network that encircles the cardiac *onlage* in very early embryonic life.

Other references bearing on the subjects in this plate are as follows: Pulmonary veins enter coronary sinus: D. Nabarro, *J. Anat. and Path.*, 1902–03, **37**: 383. Persistent left superior vena cava entering coronary sinus in complete absence of right: S. A. Habershon, *Tr. Path. Soc. Lond.*, 1876, **27**: 79; A. Dietrich, *Virch. Arch.*, 1913, **212**: 119; H. Schultz, *Virch. Arch.*, 1914, **216**: 35; Gruber, *Virch. Arch.*, 1885, **99**: 492 (see also Pl. XXIV, Fig. 7, and Pl. XXV, Fig. 2c).

Fig. 1.—Both pulmonary veins empty into coronary sinus as common trunk. Patent foramen ovale.

a. Anterior view, showing interior of the greatly dilated and hypertrophied right auricle and ventricle, the huge orifice of the coronary sinus 1.8 cm. across and the patent foramen. The right chambers occupied the entire anterior aspect of the heart, the pulmonary artery was greatly dilated, the left ventricle was small and the aorta hypoplasic.

b. Posterior view, showing entrance of left into right pulmonary vein and of this into the hugely dilated coronary sinus. In this remarkable case the pulmonary veins had retained their primary connection with the sinus venosus as represented by the coronary sinus (see above), and the entire volume of aerated blood passed into the right auricle and thence, mixed with venous blood from the great veins, through the foramen ovale to the systemic circulation, a venous-arterial shunt existing (Group III). The subject was a female child aged 2 years 4½ months, with precordial bulging and systolic murmur and thrill, maximum at the fourth left interspace, who presented no cyanosis at birth but developed paroxysmal attacks at 9 months and profound terminal cyanosis 5 days before death. (From an unpublished case in the service of A. F. deGroat and Harvey Thatcher, Little Rock, Ark.* The only other case on record was reported by Nabarro, *l.c.* above.)

Fig. 2.—Anomalous communication of right coronary artery with coronary sinus by arterio-venous anastomotic loop with cirsoid aneurysmal dilatation of arterial trunk. The vessels in the coronary sulcus have been dissected out and extended. The right coronary artery expands immediately after its origin from the right aortic sinus of Valsalva into a series of huge vascular loops, atheromatous at the kinks, which projected wormlike above the epi-

cardial fat, and passed backward to the level of the posterior longitudinal sinus, where it emptied by an opening 5 mm. across into a thinner walled arterio-venous loop with convexity to the left, which encircled and opened into the lower border of the greatly dilated coronary sinus. This structure measured 2.5 cm. across and received also the dilated vena cava magna behind and the tiny oblique vein of Marshall above before emptying into the right auricle by a small orifice 3 mm. in diameter. Thebesian valve absent. The left coronary artery (seen at extreme left) was slightly dilated and atheromatous, but otherwise normal.

From a man aged 54, dying from carcinoma of pylorus, who presented no clinical manifestations of cardiac disorder. The heart was hypertrophied and subepicardial fat increased. (Reported by Bela Halpert, *Heart*, 1930, **15**: 129, and published by his permission from the original drawings.)

Fig. 3.—Persistent left superior cava emptying into the greatly dilated coronary sinus with absence of right superior cava.*

a. Anterior view, showing the large anomalous trunk coursing down from above and merging with the greatly dilated coronary sinus.

b. Interior of right auricle, showing huge mouth of coronary sinus 4 cm. in diameter and absence of all trace of orifice of right superior cava.

c. Interior of left auricle showing closed foramen ovale and entrance of pulmonary veins.

From a man aged 23, who died of cerebral abscess following staphylococcus sinusitis. No cardiac symptoms or other anomalies. (From an unpublished case in the service of Lt. Col. Foucar, Walter Reed Hospital, Washington, D. C.)

* Specimen in the Cardiac Anomaly Collection of McGill University.

PLATE XII.   ANOMALIES OF CORONARY SINUS

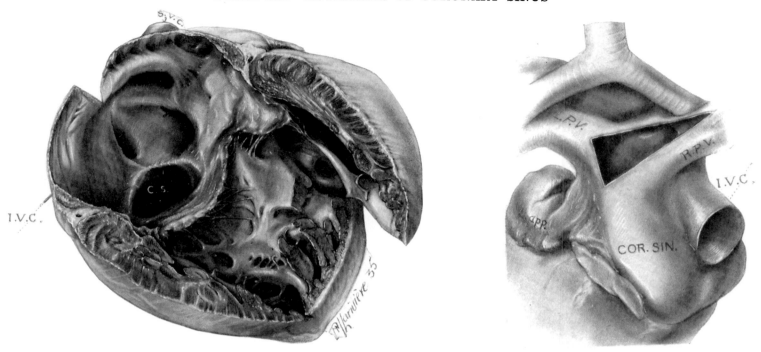

Fig. 1a.

Fig. 1b.

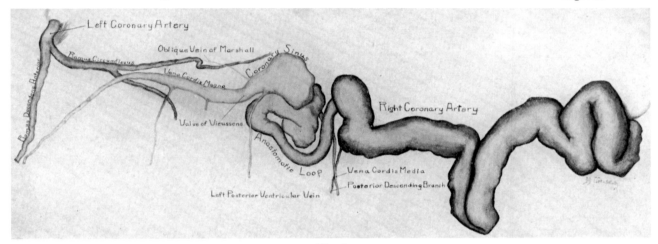

Fig. 2.

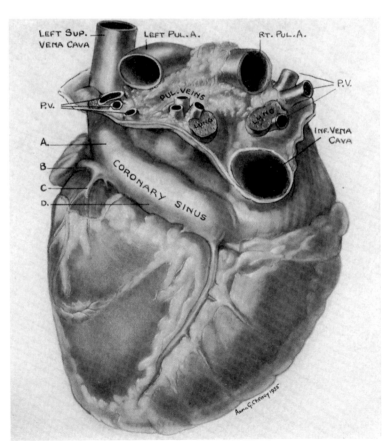

Fig. 3a.

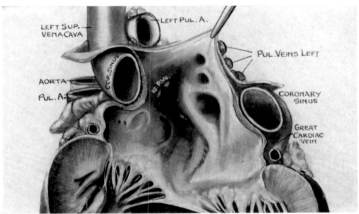

Fig. 3b.

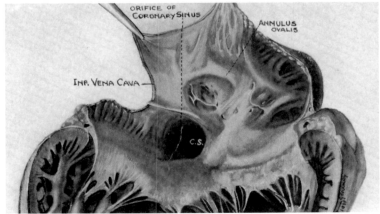

Fig. 3c.

GROUP II
CASES OF ARTERIAL-VENOUS SHUNT WITH TERMINAL REVERSAL OF FLOW
(CYANOSE TARDIVE)

PLATE XIII

PATENT DUCTUS ARTERIOSUS

In persistent patency of the ductus arteriosus it is generally assumed that a continuous leakage takes place from the aorta (in which the pressure is normally much higher than in the pulmonary artery) into the latter, an *arterial-venous shunt* existing; and that these relative pressures are maintained, in spite of the open communication between the two circulations, until some cause for respiratory obstruction sets in, such as long-continued crying, spasmodic coughing, etc., which raises the pressure in the pulmonary circulation and causes a *temporary reversal of flow* through the canal with the sudden appearance of a *transient cyanosis*, which passes off with the exciting cause. *Absence of cyanosis* except as a transient or terminal phenomenon is therefore the characteristic clinical picture of these subjects, who usually present a tall slender build and tendency to pallor significant of aortic hypoplasia. The converse may, however, be true, for in some cases fluctuation in the intra-arterial pressures seems to occur very readily, so that oxygen unsaturation of the circulating blood is raised close to its threshold value and the subjects may be of a rather stocky build with high-colored complexion and a bluish tinge of the lips on slight exertion. That the course of the blood is from left to right through the canal under otherwise normal conditions is evident from the pathology of these cases, for the pulmonary artery is practically always dilated and the left ventricle is usually hypertrophied more than the right. Moreover, in the infective processes that so frequently supervene (Fig. 4*b*) the pulmonary end of the ductus with the immediately adjacent tissues is always the initial seat of the vegetative inflammatory lesion, a very suggestive feature, as indicating that this point has been the seat of strain in the continuous passage of a left to right shunt through the defect. Characteristic physical signs are usually present, but vary according to the length of the canal and the shape of its aortic orifice. The familiar train-in-a-tunnel machinery murmur, beginning just after the first sound and continuous throughout the greater part of the cardiac cycle, localized over the first, second and third interspaces with maximum intensity at the second, with accompanying systolic or continuous thrill, which when present is pathognomonic, occurs in only about a third of the cases. In a number of others it is replaced by a double murmur of which the systolic element is apparently generated at the ductus, but the diastolic is probably that of a pulmonary insufficiency (Laubry and Pezzi). In over 30 per cent of the 92 cases analyzed by the writer, the murmur was systolic in rhythm but usually began just after the first sound, was of rather harsh character prolonged throughout systole, and of somewhat irregular localization with maximum intensity at the pulmonary area or lower over the precordium, even in some cases at the apex. A systolic murmur appears to be the rule in infants and very young children, in whom a continuous murmur is rare. Pulmonary accentuation is usually present. Other confirmatory signs are figured opposite.

Fig. 1.—Diagram by W. T. Dawson showing the course of the normal circulation after the ductus arteriosus has closed in postnatal life. The venous and arterial circulations are here entirely separate. (From Abbott and Dawson, *Internat. Clin.*, 1924, **4**: 162.)

Fig. 2.—The same, showing the foetal circulation. Here the ductus is open and, the pressure being highest in the right heart, the venous blood passes from it into the pulmonary artery and thence through the patent ductus into the descending aorta to the lower extremities, a venous-arterial shunt existing. (From Abbott and Dawson, *l.c.*)

Fig. 3.—The same, showing the circulation in persistent patency of the ductus. The pressure being highest in postnatal life on the systemic side, oxygenated blood passes from the aorta through its open lumen into the pulmonary artery, *an arterial-venous shunt existing* (shown by black arrow), until such time as a change in the relative pressures sets in, when *a reversal of flow* takes place (shown by the broken arrow) and venous blood flows into the arterial stream. (From Abbott and Dawson, *l.c.*)

Fig. 4.—Patent ductus arteriosus with acute infective endocarditis originating at pulmonary end of ductus, mycotic aneurysm of pulmonary artery and embolic abscesses in the lungs in pneumococcus septicaemia.
a. The thoracic aorta laid open from behind to show the widely patent ductus admitting a penhandle, and slight coarctation of the descending arch.
b. Heart and lungs laid open to show the interior of the right ventricle and the greatly dilated pulmonary artery of the right lung. The latter is riddled with abscess cavities, and the pulmonary lumen is occupied by a huge thrombotic mass of vegetations which block the orifice of the ductus and extend downward toward the pulmonary cusps, which are free and healthy. The aorta (seen extended above) is hypoplasic.
From a slender delicately built girl of 19 who presented a continuous machinery murmur with systolic accentuation and thrill with maximum intensity in the second left interspace, x-ray cap and "Gerhardt" dullness without

any sign of valvular disease, and who died after some weeks of great prostration, chills and septic temperature with pneumococci in the blood stream. Both the patency and the location of the infective process were diagnosed intra vitam from the classic picture presented. Microscopic examination showed the initial lesion situate at the pulmonary orifice of the ductus and extending along its lumen and that of the pulmonary artery with abundant pneumococci in the vegetations and in the embolic infarcts in the lungs. (Reported by W. F. Hamilton and M. E. Abbott, *Tr. Assn. Amer. Phys.*, 1914, **29**: 294. Drawing of Fig. *b* above by J. H. Atkinson from the specimen in the Cardiac Anomaly Collection of McGill University.)

Fig. 5.—Roentgenograph of the heart in a case of patent ductus, showing large pulmonary arc (x-ray cap), widening of pulmonary vessels at hilum and hypertrophy of both sides of the heart. The patient was a woman of 26 who presented the classic physical signs of this lesion and *complete paralysis of the left recurrent laryngeal nerve* from pressure upon this of the dilated ductus. Diagnosis made during life by W. S. Thayer. Death from multiple ruptures of the right ventricle. (Reported by Kate C. Mead, *J.A.M.A.*, 1910, **55**: 2205. Republished by permission.)

Fig. 6.—Heart-signs record from a case of patent ductus with continuous, murmur, showing low-pitched character, systolic and diastolic accentuation area of maximum intensity, zone of transmission, and variation at different areas of the precordium, in the dorsal recumbent, lateral recumbent and sitting postures, with point of maximum intensity of accompanying thrill. (Original diagram made for this Atlas by H. N. Segall. See his articles, *Amer. Heart J.*, 1933, **8**: 533; *Canad. Med. Assn. J.*, 1932, **27**: 632.)

Fig. 7.—Electrocardiogram from a case of patent ductus **showing normal curves.** (From *Clinical Electrocardiography* by Sir Thomas Lewis, 1934.)

Fig 8.—Orthodiagraphic tracings from six cases of patent ductus, showing enlarged pulmonary arc (x-ray cap of Zinn) and cardiac enlargement. (From Th. and F. M. Groedel, *Deutsch. Arch. f. klin. Med.*, 1911.)

PLATE XIII. PATENT DUCTUS ARTERIOSUS

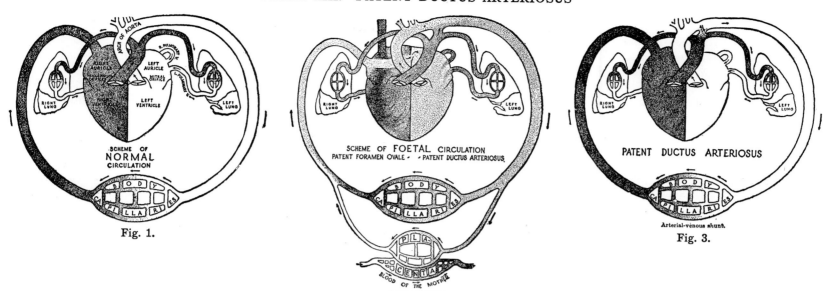

Fig. 1.

Fig. 2.

Fig. 3.

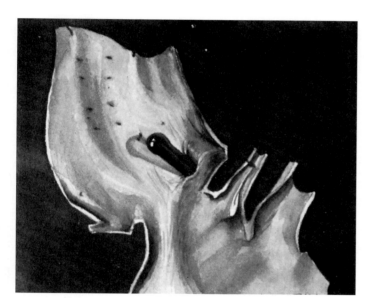

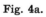

Fig. 4a.

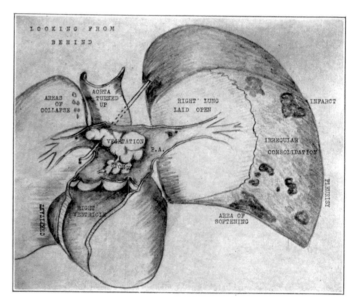

Fig. 4b.

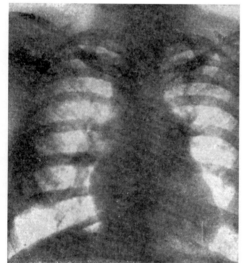

Fig. 5.

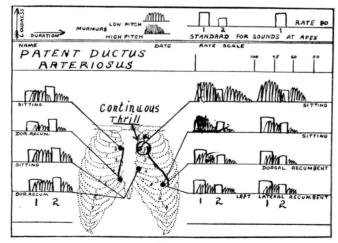

Fig. 6.

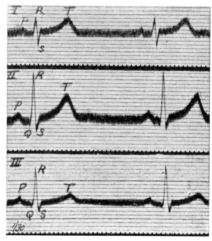

Fig. 7.

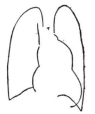

Fig. 8a.

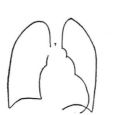

Fig. 8b.

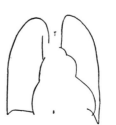

Fig. 8c.

PLATE XIV

DEFECTS OF THE INTERAURICULAR SEPTUM AND PATENT FORAMEN OVALE

These cases may be divided, from the clinical standpoint, and for convenience of discussion, into two main categories, which are illustrated by the diagrams opposite, namely, defects at the upper part of the interauricular septum, with which are included cases of primary persistent patency of the foramen ovale (Figs. 1–5), and defects at the lower part of this (persistent ostium primum Figs. 6–8). The latter cases are always associated with cleavage and insufficiency of the anterior mitral segment, and so do not produce a distinctive clinical picture but are of especial interest from their frequent association with mongolian idiocy (Fig. 8). Large defects at the upper part of this septum, on the other hand, are among the most interesting and significant chapters in the entire range of congenital cardiac disease. For these cases demonstrate, more conclusively than any others of the *cyanose tardive* group, the dynamic effects of a persistent arterial-venous shunt upon the heart and circulation. Moreover, they supply, in the great dilatation of the pulmonary artery and the eccentric hypertrophy of the heart with hypoplasia of the aorta that invariably supervene, direct anatomical proof that the course of the anomalous current is from left to right through the defect until such time as a failing left heart induces a reversal of flow with signs of congestive failure and the sudden onset of a "late cyanosis." A classic example of this type is shown in Fig. 2. So pronounced are the changes in all cases of large auricular septal defects that a definite clinical entity is established, which can be diagnosed with a fair degree of certainty in the light of modern roentgenological findings, especially in cases in which physical signs of the defect are localized over the midprecordium or midsternum, and a venous pulse is perceptible in the neck and liver. H. Roesler (*Arch. Int. Med.*, 1934, **54**: 339) points out that, in the cases of massive right-sided cardiac enlargement in which dilatation predominates over hypertrophy, the silhouette of the right heart as seen by x-rays extends usually far into the left chest with the huge pulmonary arc above on the left and the aortic knob diminished or absent; and that for the same reason the electrocardiogram shows only a *moderate* right predominance in the presence of extreme right heart enlargement.

Acquired valvular lesions, especially mitral insufficiency and stenosis, are very commonly associated with these defects and the latter combination forms the well-recognized syndrome known as mitral stenosis with interauricular insufficiency, of which the classic example shown opposite (Fig. 5) was reported by the writer a year before Lutembacher described this condition as a clinical entity.

In two cases of paradoxical embolism through a patent foramen ovale presented by W. W. Beattie (Fig. 3), this author made the important observation that, in cases of *valvular* patency, this phenomenon can take place only when a previous pulmonary embolism has reduced the pressure in the right auricle.

(For bibliography see page 38.)

Fig. 1.—Diagram showing the course of the circulation in patent foramen ovale and defect at the upper part of the interauricular septum. The pressure being highest under physiological conditions in the left auricle, the direction of the shunt is from left to right through the defect (indicated by the solid black arrow) until a pathological rise of pressure sets in in the right auricle leading to a reversal of flow (broken arrow). (From the article by W. T. Dawson and M. E. Abbott, *Internat. Clin.*, 1924, **4**: 164, Fig. 6.)

Fig. 2.—Huge defect at upper part of interauricular septum above and posterior to closed foramen ovale. Pulmonary dilatation and atheroma with insufficiency and calcification of cusps and hypoplasia of aorta. Eccentric hypertrophy of right chambers.*

a. Left heart laid open to show: *a*, the narrow hypoplasic aorta; *b*, the cut edge of the dilated pulmonary artery; *c*, the narrow aortic vestibule; *d*, the relatively small left auricle; *e*, the auricular septal defect, size of half a dollar; *f*, the closed foramen ovale; *g*, the defective auricular septum; *h*, the mitral valve; *i*, the interior of left ventricle.

b. The greatly dilated and hypertrophied right chambers laid open to show: *a*, the huge defect in the interauricular septum; *b*, orifice of inferior vena cava; *c*, complete absence of Eustachian valve or annulis ovalis; *d*, the dilated coronary sinus; *e*, the dilated sinus of the right ventricle; *f*, orifice of superior vena cava; *g*, the defective inter-auricular septum; *h*, passage into conus of right ventricle.

c. The base of the pulmonary conus showing the greatly dilated artery with thickened, calcareous and insufficient cusps, the hypoplasic aorta and the dilated right auricle above and behind this. (Drawing by A. Cheney.)

From a woman aged 64, who had worked hard as a charwoman and had had perfect health until six months before death. Since then transient cyanosis and malaise. Admitted semicomatose with marked cyanosis and oedema and died before examination of the chest could be made. (Reported by M. E. Abbott and J. Kaufmann, *J. Path. and Bact.*, 1910, **14**: 525, Case 1.)

Fig. 3.—Widely patent foramen ovale with antemortem adherent thrombus in right auricular appendix, which became the source of paradoxical embolism. The foramen measured 3 by 2 cm. The right chambers were greatly dilated and there was a small associated defect at base of the interventricular septum. *a*, foramen ovale; *b*, auricular septum.

From a man aged 49, who became short-winded at 39 and developed deep cyanosis with oedema shortly before death from oedema of the glottis. (From W. W. Beattie, "Paradoxical embolism associated with two types of patent foramen ovale," *J. Tech. Meth.*, 1925, **11**: 64.)

Fig. 4.—Orthodiagraph from a case of mitral stenosis with patent foramen ovale, showing characteristic mitral configuration with great enlargement of pulmonary arc and right heart and absence of aortic knob. (Reported by W. Dressler and H. Roesler, *Ztsch. f. klin. Med.*, 1930, **112**: 42, Fig. 3.)

Fig. 5.—Large gaping foramen ovale with calcified lower border and fenestrated annulus ovalis and acquired button hole mitral stenosis, great dilatation and hypertrophy of right ventricle, widening of pulmonary and slight coarctation of aorta.* *a*, pocket in wall of left auricle.

From a married woman aged 38, who had borne one child. Menses set in at 21 and disappeared at 28. Acute rheumatism at 14. Repeated attacks of failing compensation since age of 28. Right hemiplegia at 30 (crossed embolism?). Admitted in congestive failure with auricular fibrillation, anasarca and severe dyspnoea. Examination showed a *presystolic murmur and faint thrill at fourth left interspace near sternum.* Terminal cyanosis. (Case of C. F. Martin. Reported by M. E. Abbott, *Int. Assn. Med. Mus. Bull.*, 1915, **5**: 129. *Also in Blumer's Bedside Diag.*, 1928, **2**: 399, Fig. 254.)

Fig. 6.—Diagram of the circulation in defect at the lower part of the interauricular septum (persistent ostium primum). The remarks made under Fig. 1 regarding the direction of shunt and terminal reversal of flow apply here also. (From Dawson and Abbott, *ibid.*, p. 165.)

Fig. 7.—Large crescentic defect at lower border of interauricular septum with cleavage of anterior mitral segment, hypertrophy and dilatation of both auricles but especially right and right ventricle, dilatation of pulmonary artery and hypoplasia of aorta.*

The heart is laid open to show the interior of the left chambers: *a*, the dilated left auricle; *b*, the two parts of the cleft anterior segment of the mitral valve; *c*, the closed foramen ovale; *d*, the auricular septal defect persistent ostium primum.

From a strong well-developed man of 35, who died of perforative appendicitis. Confused heart sounds were heard at the apex. No cyanosis. (Reported by M. E. Abbott and J. Kaufmann, *J. Path. and Bact.*, 1910, **14**: 525, Case 2.)

Fig. 8.—Persistent ostium primum with cleavage of anterior mitral segment and deformity of tricuspid septal cusp. No cyanosis.*

The auricular septum presents a valvular patency of the foramen ovale and ends below in a crescentic free border which forms the upper boundary of a defect 3 by 2 cm. large, the lower border of which is formed by the overlapping upper halves of the completely divided anterior mitral segment.

From an infant which presented a peculiar murmur over the precordium and was the subject of *mongolian idiocy.* Death at 10 months from bronchopneumonia. (Case of Keith Gordon. Reported by M. E. Abbott, *Int. Assn. Med. Mus. Bull.*, 1924, **10**: 111, Case 2.)

Fig. 9.—Premature closure of the foramen ovale with generalized anasarca of the foetus and pulmonary artery joining descending aorta through widely patent ductus.*

The valvula foraminis ovalis forms a distended membrane bulging into the left auricle and above it is seen the crescentic border of the closed foramen ovale.

From a male foetus, stillborn in the eighth month of the mother's second pregnancy, which was characterized by great hydramnios. The entire body was the seat of an enormous generalized oedema and the right auricle was distended. The foramen was seen to be occupied by a thin translucent membrane crossed by numerous fine trabeculae, which apparently closed it completely.

(From William Osler, "Cases of cardiac abnormalities," *Montreal Gen. Hosp. Clin. and Path.*, 1880, **1**: 177.)

* Specimen in the Cardiac Anomaly Collection of McGill University.

PLATE XIV. DEFECTS OF INTERAURICULAR SEPTUM AND PATENT FORAMEN OVALE

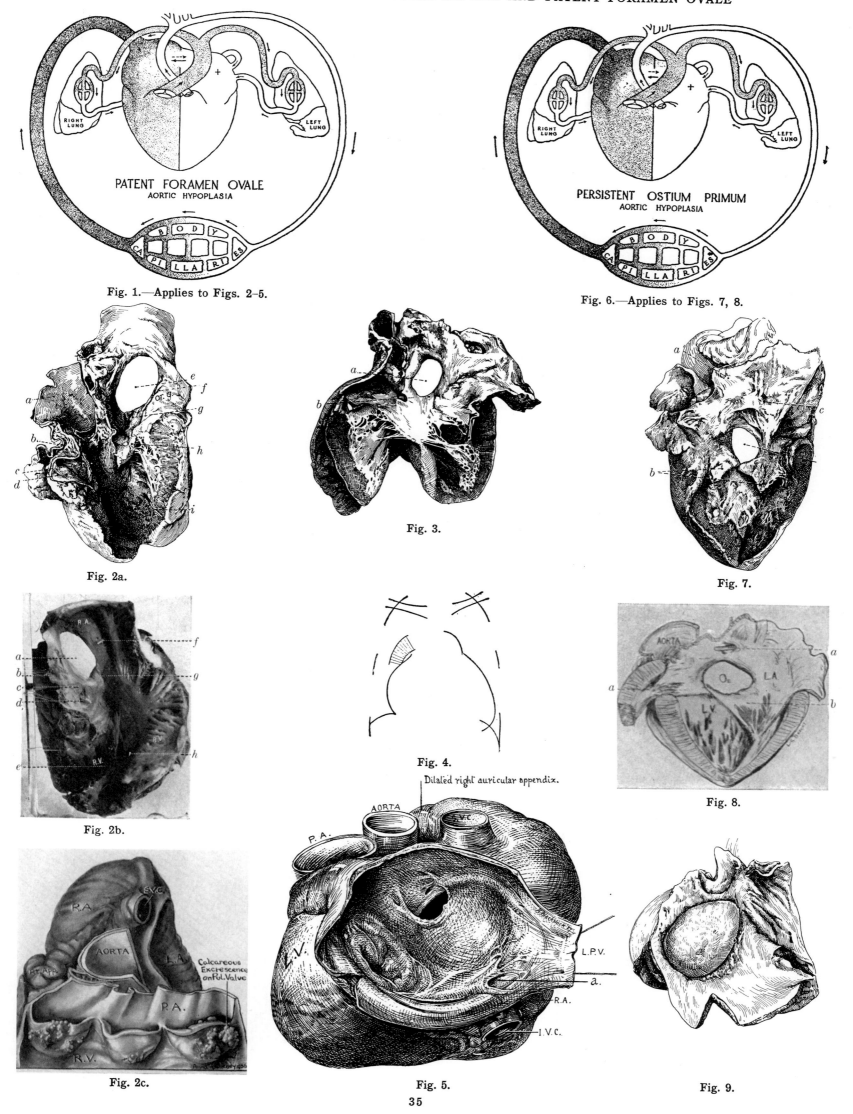

Fig. 1.—Applies to Figs. 2–5.

Fig. 6.—Applies to Figs. 7, 8.

Fig. 2a.

Fig. 3.

Fig. 7.

Fig. 2b.

Fig. 4.

Fig. 8.

Fig. 2c.

Fig. 5.

Fig. 9.

PLATE XV

A. DEFECTS OF INTERVENTRICULAR SEPTUM. B. DEFECTS OF AORTIC SEPTUM

A. Localized defects of the interventricular septum are usually situate at the base of the heart just anterior to the pars membranacea and open on the side of the right ventricle behind the septal tricuspid segment.   Less commonly the defect lies more anteriorly and opens into the conus of the right ventricle (bulbar septal defect, Fig. 9); or in a few rare instances it may lie in the lower part of the septum, as is normal in the heart of the python (Pl. III, Fig. 4), and as occurred in the remarkable case of E. Weiss (*Arch. Int. Med.*, 1927, **39** : 705). In uncomplicated cases of defects in the first of these locations (*maladie de Roger*), this is usually quite a small opening which transmits an arterial-venous shunt of blood into the right ventricle with considerable force, the current impinging upon the opposite wall of the latter and often producing there a patch of fibrosis.   Such a defect in this location has little or no effect upon the general circulation.   The physical signs, however, are usually distinctive, consisting of a holosystolic rather harsh murmur maximum in the third or fourth left interspace, accompanied in about a third of the cases by a distinct thrill (Fig. 2).   The electrocardiogram reveals in some cases a partial heart block (Fig. 7), indicating that interference with the bundle fibers has occurred.   Cyanosis is absent except as a transient or terminal feature, and is even then rare.   The clinical picture is thus that of *absence of symptoms in the presence of distinctive physical signs* in an otherwise normal individual, and the significance of this lesion lies not in the functional effect of the defect, but in the great frequency with which a subacute bacterial endocarditis develops along its margins or on the opposite wall of the right ventricle (Fig. 6).

B. Defect of the aortic septum may be located above the valves or, more commonly, it occupies the right aortic sinus of Valsalva and leads into the pulmonary conus either as a direct communication or as a thin-walled aneurysmal sac which undergoes rupture in later life (Fig. 9).   A bulbar septal defect below the aortic cusps is not infrequently associated.   The physical signs are characteristic of the arterial-venous communication above the cusps and the danger of infective endarteritis is very great.

A. See on this subject; H. Roger, "Communication congènital du coeur par inocclusion du septum interventriculaire," *Bull. de l'acad. de Méd.*, 1879, **8** : 1074; E. Dupré, *Bull. Soc. Anat. de Paris*, 1891, **5** : 404; LeHoux, "La cyanose tardive" (*maladie de Roger*), Paris Thesis, 1902; Hart, *Virch. Arch.*, 1905, Bd. 181, 57; J. G. Mönckeberg, "Ueber das Verhalten des atrio-ventriculaire System in Cortriloculare Biatriatum," *Studien z. Path., u. Entwickelung*, 1920, **2** : 448; E. Weiss, "Large defect in lower part of interventricular septum with impaired conduction and terminal cyanosis," *Arch. Int. Med.*, 1927, **39** : 705.

B. See the article by M. E. Abbott on "Clinical and developmental study of a case of ruptured aneurysm of the right anterior aortic sinus of Valsalva," *Contrib. Med. Biol. Research, Sir William Osler Anniversary Volume*, Paul B. Hoeber, 1919, **2** : 899 (Figs. 9a, b and c) for full bibliography on this subject to that date; also articles by Hektoen, "Large defect in septum between pulmonary artery and aorta, the heart normally developed.   *Tr. Path. Soc.*, Chicago, Nov. 12, 1900; C. Goehrung, *J. Med. Research*, 1920–21, **42** : 49; T. G. Moorhead and E. C. Smith, *Irish J. Med. Sci.*, 1923, p. 545, Fig. 1.

A

Fig. 1.—Diagram showing the course of the circulation in localized, uncomplicated defects at the base of the interventricular septum (maladie de Roger). The black arrow passing from left to right through the defect shows that the shunt is arterial-venous under the normal conditions of a relatively higher pressure in the left ventricle. The dotted arrow in the opposite (right to left) direction indicates the possibility of a (terminal) reversal of flow. (From Abbott and Dawson, *Internat. Clin.*, 1924, **4** : 166.)

Fig. 2.—Heart-signs record from a case of maladie de Roger. Graphic representation of the holosystolic murmur and accompanying thrill with maximum intensity at the fourth left interspace near sternal border; also variations of the murmur, in intensity, pitch and relation to first sound, at the pulmonary and aortic areas, at apex, along the right sternal border and posteriorly at left angle of scapula. (Diagram and record made for this Atlas by H. N. Segall. Reference under Pl. XIII, Fig. 6.)

Fig. 3.—Small ventricular septal defect just anterior to the undefended space (maladie de Roger), view from left ventricle.* The anomalous opening admits a knitting needle and has sclerosed thickened margins. Heart was not enlarged and weighed 230 gm. From a female aged 20, who died accidentally (from burning). Specimen 14.122² in the Medical Museum, presented by John McCrae. (Republished from the article by M. E. Abbott in *Osler's Mod. Med.*, 1927, **4** : 690, Fig. 62.)

Fig. 4.—Large ventricular defect at base admitting a slate pencil. View from right ventricle.* From an infant aged 49 days. The right ventricle was slightly hypertrophied and the pulmonary artery dilated. Specimen No. 14.122³, presented by John McCrae. (Republished, *ibid.*, p. 689, Fig. 61.)

Fig. 5.—Orthodiagraphic drawing from a young man aged 17. Diagnosed clinically as ventricular septal defect. Second (pulmonary) arc is slightly increased. Right auricular border pulsated very strongly and synchronously with left border. Ventricles slightly enlarged symmetrically. (From A. Dietlin, *Herz und Gefässe im Roentgenbild*, 1923, Fig. 115, p. 225.)

Fig. 6.—Ventricular septal defect (maladie de Roger) with acute bacterial endocarditis of tricuspid segments adjacent to and screening the defect. **Staphylococcus septicaemia.** View looking into right ventricle showing the small circular orifice of the defect, with smooth margins lying just behind the infundibular tricuspid segment, the ventricular surface and chordae tendineae of which are loaded with thrombotic vegetations. The endocardium elsewhere appears healthy. Apex slightly bifid.

From a previously healthy boy of 2½ years, who presented a moderately long, slightly harsh precordial systolic murmur, maximal to left of lower sternum attended by a systolic thrill over midsternum. No cyanosis or clubbing. Developed suddenly a severe sore throat with epistaxis and high temperature and two weeks later admitted to the Good Samaritan Hospital, Boston, in profound toxaemia, leucocytes 40,000. S. Albus in pure culture in blood stream. Diagnosis of Roger's disease with infective endocarditis made intra vitam. (Published by courtesy of Paul D. White. Art drawing made for this Atlas by Muriel McLatchie, Massachusetts General Hospital.)

* Specimen in the Cardiac Anomaly Collection of McGill University.

Fig. 7.—Electrocardiogram showing partial heart block in a case of maladie de Roger. From a boy aged 10 years. The tracing shows a sinus rhythm with a partial A-V block of 2:1 degree. The auricular rate is 78, the ventricular 38 per minute. There is no delay in bundle branch conduction or in the electrical axis deviation. The contour of the deflection is normal. (Tracing and interpretation by G. Nicolson.)

B

Fig. 8.—Diagram showing course of the circulation in defect of the aortic septum. Note that the anomalous communication between the aorta and pulmonary artery is directly above the valves and that an arterial-venous shunt (indicated by black arrow) exists. (From Abbott and Dawson, *Internat. Clin.*, 1924, **4** : 166.)

Fig. 9.—Congenital aneurysm of right aortic sinus of Valsalva rupturing into conus of right ventricle with associated bulbar septal defect and extensive subacute infective endocarditis with aortic and pulmonary insufficiency, hypoplasia of aorta and dilatation of pulmonary artery.*

a. View of interior of right ventricle showing long tubular aneurysm opening into conus just below pulmonary cusps with bulbar septal defect immediately below this, and probes passed through both orifices. Luxuriant vegetations of infective endocarditis clothing margins of the defects, opposite wall of the conus and the thickened pulmonary segments. (Drawing by J. H. Atkinson.)

b. Interior of left ventricle and aortic valve showing the probes passed through the defects in the right ventricle emerging in the sinus of Valsalva above and in base of left ventricle below the right aortic cusp, with thickening and insufficiency of all segments.

From a tall spare man aged 36, intelligence above average, in perfect health until nine years before death, when after a severe strain he suddenly developed symptoms of cardiac insufficiency, never well since. On examination, heaving precordial impulse and very superficial diastolic thrill of maximum intensity in second and third left interspaces transmitted to left midaxillary and right nipple line, and very loud rough continuous murmur with diastolic accentuation, maximum in third left interspace, heard 2 in. from chest wall and over entire thorax. Low red cell count and leucocytosis, high septic temperature with occasional chills. Slight oedema but never cyanosis. (From a case in the service of W. F. Hamilton reported by M. E. Abbott in *Contrib. to Med. and Biol. Research Sir Wm. Osler Memorial*, P. B. Hoeber, 1919, **2** : 899, Figs. 1 and 2.)

Fig. 10.—Model by Tandler showing interior of embryonic bulbus cordis at a stage when two points of communication existed between the great trunks above and below the point of fusion of the distal bulbar swellings 1 and 3. *A.*, aorta (fourth right arch); *P.*, attachment of pericardium; *Pl.*, pulmonary artery (sixth arch); *d. Bw.* 1–3, distal bulbar swellings 1 and 3; *p. Bw. A–B*, proximal bulbar swellings A and B; * point at which the sound in the common lumen disappears, and ** point at which it reappears below in the common lumen of the bulbis cordis; *S.a.p.*, septum aortico-pulmonale. Compare the defects above and below the right aortic cusp in Fig. 9b. (From Keibel and Mall, *Embryology*, 1912, **2** : 532.   Reprinted by permission.)

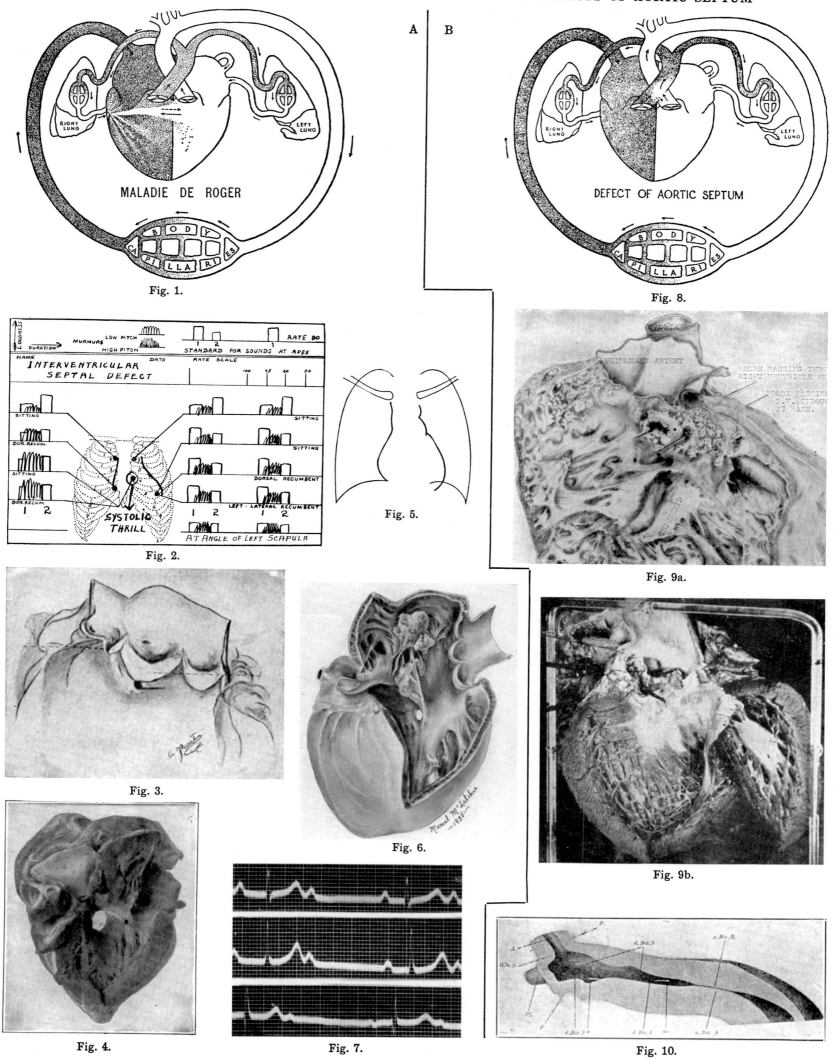

Fig. 1.

Fig. 2.

Fig. 3.

Fig. 4.

Fig. 5.

Fig. 6.

Fig. 7.

Fig. 8.

Fig. 9a.

Fig. 9b.

Fig. 10.

MISCELLANEOUS ADDITIONAL REFERENCES

PLATE XIV

In addition to the articles cited under the cases described on p. 36 see also the following: Bard and Curtillet, "Contribution a l'étude de la physiologie de la maladie bleue; forme tardive de cette affection," *Rev. de méd.*, 1889, **9**: 993; T. Thompson and W. Evans, "Paradoxical embolism," *Quart. J. Med.*, 1930, **23**: 135; R. Lutembacher, "De la stenose mitrale avec communication interauriculaire," *Arch. d. mal. du coeur*, 1916, **9**: 235; also in *Presse Med.*, 1925, p. 236; W. Dressler and H. Roesler, "Vorhofseptumdefekt Kombiniert mit Mitralstenose und aurikulärem Leberpuls," *Ztsch. f. klin. Med.*, 1930, **112**: 421; N. W. Ingalls, "Vena cava superior receiving two upper right pulmonary veins and opening into both atria," *Bull. Johns Hopkins Hosp.*, 1907, **18** No. 193; S. McGinn and P. D. White, "Interauricular septal defect associated with mitral stenosis," *Amer. Heart J.*, 1933, **9**: 1; H. Roesler, "Interatrial septal defect," *Arch. Int. Med.*, 1934, **54**: 339; E. Lehman, "Congenital atresia of the foramen ovale," *Amer. J. Dis. Child.*, 1927, **33**: 585; S. Gibson and A. Roos, "Open foramen ovale associated with mitral stenosis," *Amer. J. Dis. Child.*, 1935, **50**: 1465; H. J. Hirschboeck, "Paradoxical embolism," *Amer. J. Med. Sci.*, 1935, **189**: 236.

PLATE XXI

Persistent ostium atrio-ventriculare commune with mongolian idiocy: F. D. Gunn and J. M. Dieckmann, *Amer. J. Path.*, 1927, **3**: 595; G. M. Robson, *Amer. J. Path.*, 1931, **7**: 299; J. G. Mönckeberg, *Centr. f. allg. Path. u. path. Anat.*, 1923, **33**: 144; M. E. Abbott and K. Gordon, *J. Tech. Meth.*, 1924, **10**: 115; Cassel, *Berl. klin. Woch.*, 1917, **54**: 159; F. P. Mall, *Amer. J. Anat.*, 1912, **13**: 249; H. Schleussing, *Arch. f. klin. Med.*, 1925, **254**: 579; Dublizhaza, *Zurich Thesis*, 1906. Cor triloculare biatriatum with anomalous septum cutting off rudimentary right chamber: T. B. Peacock, *Tr. Path. Soc. Lond.*, 1855, **6**: 117; H. Chiari, *Cent. f. d. med. Wissensch.*, 1880, p. 186; J. D. Mann, *Brit. Med. J.*, 1905, **1**: 614; A. H. Young, *J. Anat. and Phys.*, 1907, **41**: 190; Marchand, *Deutsch. Path. Ges.*, 1908, **12**: 174; E. S. Mills, *J. Med. Research*, 1923, **44**: 257. With rudimentary left chamber: D. Kornblum, *Amer. J. Path.* 1935, **11**: 803, also, S. K. Ngai, *Amer. J. Path.*, 1935, **11**: 309.

PLATE XXIII

See under Pl. II, III and IV for further discussion of this subject and additional references. Also C. Rokitansky, *Die Defeckte der Scheidewände des Herzens*, Vienna, Braumüller, 1875; A. Spitzer, *Roux's Arch. f. Entwick.*, Part I, 1919, **45**: 686; *Arch. f. path. Anat.*, 1923, **243**: 81; *Ztsch. f. d. ges. Anat.* (Abt. 1), 1927, **84**: 30; K. Katsujo, *Amer. J. Dis. Child.*, 1930, **39**: 363; P. F. Shapiro, *Arch. Path.*, 1930, **9**: 54; W. Feldman and A. Chalmers, *Brit. J. Dis. Child.*, 1933, **30**: 27.

PLATE XXV

Congenital dextrocardia: S. L. Brimblecombe, *Brit. Med. J.*, 1920, **2**: 891; S. A. Reinberg and M. E. Mandelstam, *Radiology*, 1928, **11**: 240; A. Spitzer, *Virch. Arch.*, 1929, **27**: 226; H. Roesler, *Wien. Arch. f. inn. Med.*, 1930, **19**: 505; Corrected transposition: see Rokitansky, Pl. XXIII; Löchte, *Zieg. Beit.*, 1871, **24**; Tönnies, Göttingen Thesis, 1884. Congenital heart block: E. P. Carter and J. Howland, *Bull. Johns Hopkins Hosp.*, 1920, **31**: 351; P. D. White, R. S. Eustis and W. J. Kerr, *Amer. J. Dis. Child.*, 1921, **22**: 299; J. G. Wilson and R. T. Grant, *Heart*, 1926, **12**: 295; H. Davis and R. M. Stecher, *Amer. J. Dis. Child.*, 1928, **36**: 115; G. B. Fleming and M. M. Stevenson, *Arch. Dis. Child.*, 1928, **3**: 221; G. Nicolson, H. I. Shulman and D. L. Green, *Amer. J. Dis. Child.*, 1929, **37**: 580; W. M. Yater, *Amer. J. Dis. Child.*, 1929, **38**: 112; W. M. Yater, C. W. Barrier and P. E. McNabb, *Ann. Int. Med.*, 1934, **7**: 1263; W. M. Yater, W. G. Ledman and V. H. Cornell, *J.A.M.A.*, 1934, **102**: 1660.

GROUP III

CASES OF PERMANENT VENOUS-ARTERIAL SHUNT AND RETARDATION OF FLOW (CYANOTIC GROUP)

PLATE XVI

SYMPTOMATOLOGY OF CONGENITAL CYANOSIS

Congenital cyanosis, or *morbus coeruleus*, is the name given to the symptom complex which invariably develops when the oxygen unsaturation of the circulating blood is permanently raised above the "threshold value" at which this becomes perceptible in the capillaries (placed by the calculation of Lundsgaard and van Slyke at 6.7 volumes per cent). As was pointed out by these authors in their fundamental contribution to the elucidation of this subject, the reduced oxygenation of the blood and corresponding cyanotic hue are the result of various "influencing" and "modifying" factors, the most powerful of these in this condition being a permanent venous-arterial shunt through the defect and a retardation of flow in the capillaries (Lundsgaard's *alpha* and *D* factors, Fig. 8B), which act singly, or in combination with each other or with other elements, to produce the cyanosis of congenital heart disease. For a clear understanding of the clinical features presented, however, it is essential to remember that all such factors have been in operation from very early intrauterine life, and by their continuous action lead inevitably to capillary changes that must have an important bearing upon the peculiar symptomatology of this condition, which develops as life proceeds and serves to distinguish it from the cyanosis of acquired heart disease. Redisch and Roesler in their valuable differential study by the capillary microscope of the skin changes in these two sets of cases establish a definite histological picture of each (Figs. 4, 6) and express the belief, as does Wollheim, that the dilatation, stasis, congestion and abundant neoformation of capillaries shown in congenital cyanosis are themselves the dominating factor in the production of its symptomatology. These authors, moreover, make the pregnant suggestion that the *absence of oedema*, which is such a striking feature of the advanced stages of *morbus coeruleus*, may perhaps be explained by the above changes in the capillary loops, the skin acting by means of these expanded thick-walled channels of the subpapillary plexus as a reservoir for the stagnating and retarded blood. Certainly these patients, especially persons who have attained early adult life, and in whom therefore these insidious capillary changes have been in operation over many years, present the hallmarks of deficient oxygenation in a form that is significant of a predominating capillary factor, and that is in sharp contrast to the cyanosis seen in the last stages of cardiac decompensation. The bluish-violet discoloration of the skin and mucous membranes, deepening on slight muscular exertion to a spectacular purplish hue, the suffused conjunctivae, clubbing of nose, fingers and toes, dyspnoea and dyspnoeic attacks, and, in advanced cases, the cyanosis retinae and polycythemia sometimes amounting to twelve or thirteen million, with absence of oedema, together present a unique clinical picture that, once seen, can never be forgotten and that is in itself pathognomonic of the underlying circulatory and structural as well as tissue change.

(See page 46 for bibliography on this subject.)

Fig. 1.—Clubbing of fingers and toes in congenital cyanosis. Note the discoloration and bulbous enlargement of terminal phalanges especially the thumbs and great toes, with broadening, shortening and convexity of the nails and thickening of nailbeds. From a cyanotic child in the Medical Service of the Montreal General Hospital. Cast made by Hortense Douglas. (Reproduced here by permission from a color print made of this, published in the writer's monograph in *Nelson's Looseleaf Med.*, 1932, **4**: Pl. II facing p. 238.)

Fig. 2.—The cyanotic facies as displayed in a highly gifted patient with the tetralogy of Fallot who survived into late middle life. This is a portrait of the notable American composer, Henry Gilbert, who presented the hallmarks of congenital cyanosis from his earliest childhood, but in spite of his crippling heart condition led an active artistic life and made an important contribution to contemporary music. Examination 14 months before death showed a rather florid cyanosis, with marked clubbing of the extremities and dyspnoea on exertion, eyes alert but somewhat suffused, sight excellent. A loud blowing systolic murmur maximal at the left fourth interspace not transmitted into back or neck vessels with slight accompanying thrill. Red cells 7,700,000. Death followed 8 days after onset of left haemiplegia. At autopsy the right ventricle was greatly hypertrophied and there was a huge circular defect 2 cm. across, above which the large aorta arose dextroposed from both ventricles. Pulmonary artery bicuspid and hypoplasic and emerged anteriorly and to the left from stenosed infundibulum. (From Paul D. White and Howard Sprague, "The Tetralogy of Fallot. Report of a case in a noted musician who lived until his 60th year," *J.A.M.A.*, 1929, **92**: 787.)

Fig. 3.—Cyanosis retinae. Painting by H. Blackstock of this condition in a cyanotic boy aged $3\frac{1}{2}$ years. (Reproduced by permission from a color print published by W. B. Saunders Company in the writer's article in *Blumer's Bedside Diag.*, 1928, **2**: Fig. 311.)

Fig. 4.—Pathological changes in the capillaries in the cyanosis of decompensation in acquired heart disease (capillary microscope). From the article by Redisch and Roesler, see Fig. 6.)

Fig. 5.—Capillaries of the nailbeds seen under the microscope in a case of congenital cyanosis. Note the tortuosity and thickening of both venous and arterial ends of the capillary loops and their proximity to each other owing to formation of new capillaries. From a cyanotic girl of 12 with the tetralogy of Fallot and dying of subacute bacterial endocarditis of all valves. (Reported by S. D. Leader and M. A. Kugel, *J. Pedriat.*, 1934, **4**: 595.)

Fig. 6.—Pathological changes in the capillaries in congenital cyanosis as seen under the capillary microscope. The capillary loops show great thickening especially of their venous ends, involving their convexity and sometimes

their arterial part, and are twisted upon themselves and crowded together owing to the presence of many new formed anastomotic twigs, the whole presenting a marked contrast to that in the pathological capillary picture of acquired heart disease shown in Fig. 4 above. (From Redisch and Roesler, "Kapillarstudien," *Wien. Arch. f. inn. Med.*, 1929, **16**: 463.)

Fig. 7.—Diagrams by Lundsgaard and van Slyke showing graphically the circulation under normal conditions and under the effect of the different "influencing factors" that produce cyanosis.

a. The circulation in normal resting individuals, when the blood leaves the lungs 0.95 per cent or 19 volumes per cent saturated (indicated by stippled area) and 0.5 or 1 volume per cent oxygen unsaturated.

b. In a case of incomplete aeration in the lungs due to pneumonic consolidation, lowered oxygen tension, etc., showing the blood emerging from these incompletely saturated (*l* factor).

c. In a case of venous-arterial shunt where the blood passes from right to left through a cardiac septal defect and venous blood enters the arterial stream (*alpha factor*).

d. In a case of retardation of flow where deoxygenation is abnormally high in the peripheral capillaries at various parts of the surface of the body. (*D* factor.)

Fig. 8.—A. Diagram showing the influence on C, the mean capillary oxygen unsaturation, of T, the variations in the total oxygen combining power of the blood: of *D*, the oxidation rate during the passage of blood through the capillaries; of λ, the fraction of total haemoglobin passing unoxygenated through unaerated parts of the lungs; and of α, the fraction of venous blood passing unaerated through a cardiac defect into the arterial stream. Note that normal value of oxygen unsaturation in the capillaries is here shown to be 3.5 volumes per cent, and that the threshold value at which raised oxygen unsaturation becomes visible is 6.7 volumes per cent.

B. Diagram showing the influence on C, mean capillary oxygen unsaturation, of simultaneous variations in D and α (the two factors that commonly act in combination in the graver cases of congenital cyanosis). (From C. Lundsgaard and D. D. van Slyke, "Cyanosis" *Medicine*, 1923, **2**: 1, Figs. 12–16, 18. Reproduced by permission.)

NOTE TO READER: For the clear understanding of these important diagrams these authors' original monograph should be consulted, or the writer's discussion of this in *Blumer's Bedside Diag.*, 1928, **2**: 438–448.)

Fig. 9.—Electrocardiogram from the cyanotic patient with tetralogy of Fallot shown in Fig. 2, taken March 8, 1927. Leads I, II and III, normal rhythm, rate 66; right axis deviation, index −18, angle +140 degrees. *P* wave, lead II, 5 mm. amplitude, 0.15 second duration. Diphasic *T* wave in all leads. (From the article by P. D. White and H. B. Sprague, *J.A.M.A.*, 1929, **92**: 787, Fig. 2.)

PLATE XVI. SYMPTOMATOLOGY OF CONGENITAL CYANOSIS

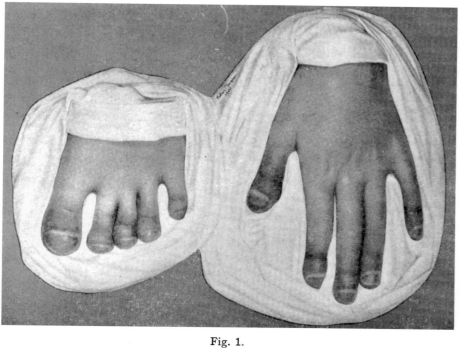

Fig. 1.

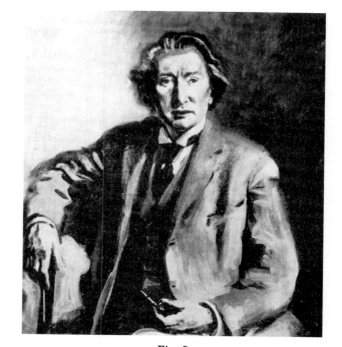

Fig. 2.

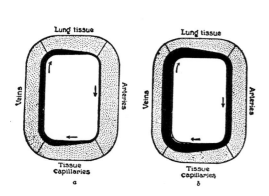

Fig. 3.

Fig. 4.

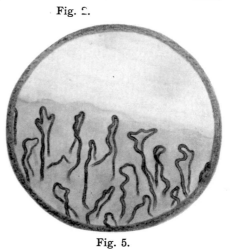

Fig. 5.

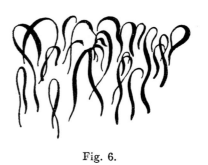

Fig. 6.

Usual threshold value of C for appearance of cyanosis. According to variations in what we term modifying factors this threshold value can be higher or lower.

Usual normal values. Brackets indicate variations ordinarily found in normal conditions.

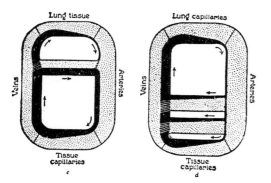

Fractional total hemoglobin in reduced form
Fractional total hemoglobin in oxygenated form

Fig. 7.

Reduced hemoglobin passing from the veins to the arteries through unaerated parts of lungs or defective heart without traversing the lungs.

Usual threshold for production of cyanosis.

Reduced hemoglobin formed by deoxydation of blood as it passes through the tissue capillaries (D).

Hemoglobin passing in reduced form from veins to arteries through aerated parts of the lungs (λ = 0.05).

Fig. 8.

Fig. 9.

41

PLATE XVII

PULMONARY CONUS STENOSIS AT LOWER BULBAR ORIFICE

ALL CARDIA SEPTA CLOSED

The two cases figured opposite are examples of that relatively small group in which retardation of flow leading to stasis and increased deoxygenation in the capillaries (Lundsgaard's *D* factor), without any complicating venous-arterial (*alpha*) shunt, was apparently the sole cause of the congenital cyanosis that existed. These cases are, however, remarkable in that the seat of the stenosis was not at the pulmonary valve but some distance below this at the "lower bulbar orifice" forming a capacious separate chamber with a small orifice in its floor. In Case 2, two such openings existed, which were the sole means of transit of the venous blood to the lungs, both foramen ovale and ductus arteriosus as well as the interventricular septum being completely closed. In both cases, cyanosis was moderate and came on late in life, in Case 2 associated with great oedema.

Stenosis of the pulmonary conus at the lower bulbar orifice, the conus a separate chamber above this, is a well-recognized form of developmental pulmonary stenosis and was reported upon by Sir Arthur Keith as a remarkable illustration of persistence of the reptilian bulbus in the adult human heart. In all the cases described by him, however, and so far as we know in the literature, except the two presented here and two reported by Lafitte (*Bull. de la soc. anat. de Paris*, 1892, **6**: 13) and Jackson (*Tr. Path. Soc. Lond.*, 1893, **44** : 29) a large ventricular septal defect was associated with some dextroposition of the aorta. In the first case shown opposite (Fig. 1) the heart was otherwise normal, but the margins of the constriction were fibrosed and the seat of luxuriant recent vegetations. In the second case (Figs. 4–8) the heart was the seat of several minor associated anomalies, including a slight dextroposition of the aorta, which was of interest as bringing it within the range of Spitzer's theory. A point of great importance in this second case was the extraordinary fibrosis and degeneration of the myocardium of the right ventricle present (Fig. 8), which was ascribed by the authors to the tremendous intraventricular pressure that must have existed behind the stenosed orifice in the presence of closure of all the foetal passages. In curious contrast to this was the complete absence of such myocardial changes in the first case (Fig. 1) under apparently the same dynamic conditions, for the foramen ovale here was also closed. (The writer takes this opportunity of correcting a mistake in the published report of this latter (Thalheimer) case to the effect that the foramen ovale *was patent*. See reference under Fig. 1.)

Fig. 1.—Stenosis of pulmonary conus at lower bulbar orifice with ventricular septum and foramen ovale closed. Subacute bacterial endocarditis of pulmonary cusps and margins of conus orifice.* S. viridans infection, embolic glomerulonephritis.

A heart laid open to show the interior of the pulmonary conus. The pulmonary artery is large and is supplied with three well-developed cusps, all of which carried polypoid vegetations, one being 1.5 cm. long and hanging free in the lumen of the artery. Below the pulmonary ring the conus cavity, 3 cm. deep with muscular walls, tapers to the slitlike opening in its floor, which is surrounded also by large vegetations. From a young married woman with a history of mental and nervous disease in sibs, who presented signs of heart disease from childhood and a very loud systolic blow maximum over the pulmonary area, but who went through two pregnancies successfully and was delivered of two normal children. Dyspnoea on exertion with occasional fainting spells and moderate cyanosis developed in recent years but no clubbing. Death followed septicaemia with infective endocarditis of the pulmonary valve and conus and sero-fibrinous pericarditis. Microscopic examination showed marked hyperplasia of muscle fibers of right ventricle but no areas of fibrosis or marked changes in blood vessels. (From the service of Wm. Thalheimer and H. A. Holbrook of Milwaukee, Wis. Specimen No. 14.131⁵ in the Cardiac Anomaly collection of McGill University. Reported by W. W. Eakin and M. E. Abbott, *Amer. J. Med. Sci.*, 1933, **186**: 860.)

Fig. 2.—Diagram of the course of the circulation in pulmonary stenosis with all cardia septa closed.

Fig. 3.—X-ray of heart of Case 1 (Fig. 1), showing widening in region of right auricle, small aortic knob and some enlargement in region of pulmonary conus.

Fig. 4.—Lateral view of head of Case 2 showing vestigial remains of left external ear, low growth of hair on neck and facial expression of mental deficiency. Note also slitlike opening for external ear, and displaced cartilaginous nodule at tip of mastoid.

Fig. 5.—Roentgenograph of heart of Case 2 (Fig. 7), showing enormous increase in transverse diameter, right border of shadow formed by dilated right auricle and left by greatly hypertrophied right ventricle, the latter extending almost to the left axillary border. Also broadening of shadow at the base on the right suggesting dilatation of the superior cava, and marked prominence of pulmonary arc on left border (*A*) due to dilated pulmonary conus. Aortic knob also prominent.

Fig. 6.—Electrocardiogram from this case showing right axis deviation and increased amplitude of *Q R S* deflections. Large *P* deflections are seen in leads I and II. The *P–R* interval is 0.24 seconds.

Fig. 7.—Stenosis of pulmonary conus at lower bulbar orifice with complete closure of all foetal passages.*

Anterior view of heart of Case 2 showing relations of great vessels at the base and conus of right ventricle laid open. Note thickened endocardium lining triangular cavity and minute conus orifices communicating with sinus of ventricle, also hypoplasia of pulmonary valve and trunk and dilated ascending aorta.

b. Interior of aortic vestibule. Note slight dextroposition of aorta and aneurysmal pars membranacea.

c. Right chambers laid open to show interior of sinus portion of right ventricle. Note massive simple hypertrophy of right ventricle and minute conus orifices, also anomalous chordae in right auricle. (Drawing from specimen No. 14.132⁵ by H. Blackstock, Medical Art Department, McGill University.)

Fig. 8.—Microphotographs from sections through myocardium of the right ventricle below stenosed bulbar orifice in this case, showing diffuse myocardial fibrosis and sclerosis of vessels with intimal hyperplasia. Upper: Mallory phosphotungstic acid. Lower: Elastic tissue stain.

From a boy aged 14 with moderate cyanosis and dyspnoea from infancy and great anasarca of entire body in later months of life, who presented a congenital papilloma of right conjunctiva, bilateral cleft of the hard palate and congenital absence of both ears, marked increase of venous pressure, pronounced systolic thrill over midprecordium and a loud blowing systolic murmur maximum at fourth left interspace. No polycythaemia until shortly before his sudden death from circulatory failure when the red count was 5,500,000. (From a case in the Children's Memorial Hospital, Montreal, reported by W. W. Eakin and M. E. Abbott, *Amer. J. Med. Sci.* 1933, **186**: 860.)

*Specimen in the Cardiac Anomaly Collection of McGill University.

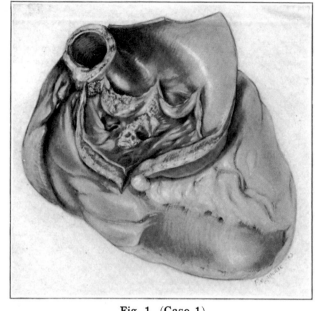

Fig. 1. (Case 1)

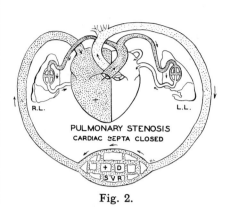

Fig. 2.

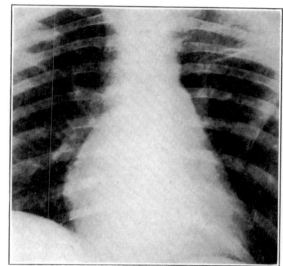

Fig. 3.

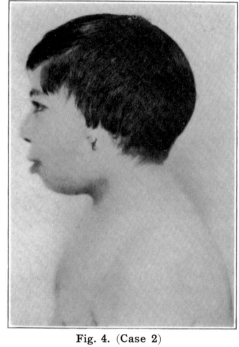

Fig. 4. (Case 2)

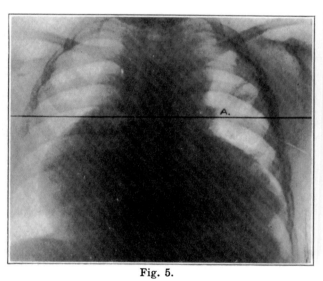

Fig. 5.

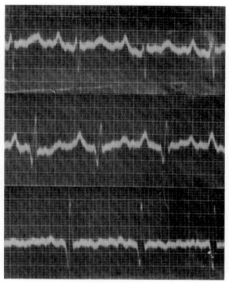

Fig. 6.

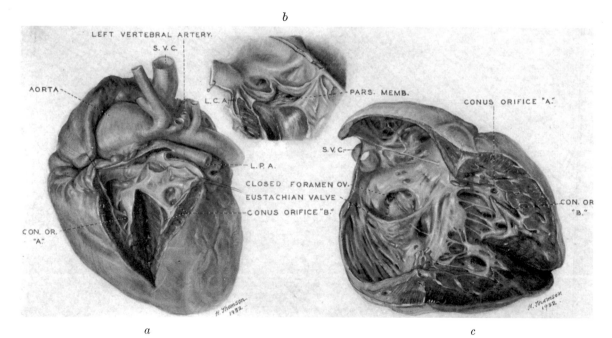

Fig. 7.

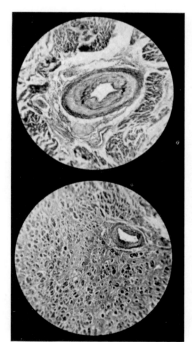

Fig. 8.

43

PLATE XVIII

A. PULMONARY AND TRICUSPID STENOSIS WITH CLOSED VENTRICULAR SEPTUM. B. EISENMENGER COMPLEX

A. Pulmonary Stenosis with Closed Septum. Apart from the rare condition of constriction at the lower bulbar orifice with all cardiac septa closed presented in Plate XVII, a group of cases exists of *valvular* pulmonary stenosis without any other complicating lesions, except, in most instances, a patent foramen ovale. This condition is practically always inflammatory, the result of an endocarditis running its course in later foetal life after septation has been completed. In these uncomplicated cases the right ventricle is always the seat of a marked simple hypertrophy and the right auricle dilated (Fig. 2), but the heart is otherwise normal. The tricuspid orifice is liable to be involved in a similar lesion of inflammatory origin (Figs. 3 and 5). Such cases are much less frequent than the developmental type of pulmonary stenosis with associated ventricular septal defect and dextroposition of the aorta (Pl. XIX), but the circulatory conditions are more favorable, in that the chief (and with closed foramen ovale, the only) cause of raised oxygen-unsaturation is retardation of flow with increased deoxygenation in the capillaries (Lundsgaard's D factor), a venous-arterial shunt (l factor) being either absent, or (where the foramen ovale is open) present in a much smaller volume than in the large shunt that takes place through an associated septal defect in the so-called "tetralogy of Fallot" (Pl. XIX). Cyanosis is therefore usually moderate in degree and of relatively late onset, frequently not appearing until after early childhood. The condition tends, too, to become progressive, though recurrent attacks of rheumatic endocarditis upon the thickened valve are a common event. This is well illustrated in the classic case shown in Fig. 6, in which cyanosis first appeared in the ninth year. Clubbing became however, a very marked feature, the capillary factor evidently predominating. For the same reason the average duration of life is longer than in the tetralogy, although Paul White's famous musician (Pl. XVII), who presented a classic example of the latter combination, broke the record for both groups by surviving into his sixtieth year. Because of the superficial location of the lesion and of the fact that the current is not deflected into the aorta through a septal defect, physical signs, consisting of a harsh systolic murmur with a pronounced thrill, maximum at the pulmonary area, are usually very marked. There may be an enlarged pulmonary arc from dilatation of the pulmonary trunk above the valve; and right predominance is a marked feature of the electrocardiogram.

B. Eisenmenger Complex. This term has been used by the writer, in default of a better, to designate an unusual combination, which was first diagnosed during life by von Schrötter and was reported by Eisenmenger (*Ztsch. f. klin. Med.*, 1897, **32**: 1), of ventricular septal defect with dextroposition of the aorta without any pulmonary stenosis or hypoplasia. This rare condition is to be distinguished from the much more frequent tetralogy of Fallot, in which pulmonary stenosis is an essential feature of the otherwise identical combination. The term "biventricular aorta" has been proposed by Blackford for those cases of *reitende aorta* in which this vessel rides astride the septum arising from both ventricles above the defect, but it does not cover others in which it springs "dextroposed" entirely from the right ventricle. As both these types form a single clinical group, we are still in need of a generic name, if that adopted by the writer is discarded. Cyanosis and clubbing in these cases are moderate and set in late and the latter feature may be absent. Physical signs are those of the septal defect, and the systolic murmur is usually heard in the back but not in the vessels of the neck. A classic example of this condition in a man aged 60 years with atheroma of the dilated pulmonary artery and calcification and insufficiency of the pulmonary valve has been reported lately by H. L. Stewart and B. L. Crawford (*Amer. J. Path.*, 1933, **9**: 637).

A

Fig. 1.—Diagram of the circulation in pulmonary stenosis with closed ventricular septum and patent foramen ovale. (From Abbott and Dawson, *Internat. Clin.*, 1924, **4**: 172, Fig. 11.)

Fig. 2.—Heart showing pulmonary stenosis from inflammatory fusion of cusps: ventricular septum closed. A classic example of this condition in an adult heart. The right ventricle is hypertrophied and the right auricle greatly dilated. (Reproduced by permission from "Les affections congénitales" by J. Fleury in *Encyclopédie Medico-Chirurgicale*, 1934, **12**: 4075, Fig. 293.)

Fig. 3.—Pulmonary and tricuspid stenosis of inflammatory origin—ventricular septum closed.* Great hypertrophy of right ventricle and dilatation of right auricle. Male infant aged 4 months. Moderate cyanosis becoming extreme before death from bronchitis, small patency of foramen ovale. (Reported by Wm. Osler, *Montreal Gen. Hosp. Repts. Clin. and Path.*, 1880, **1**: 185, Pl. IV, Figs. 1, 2. Specimen No. 7422 in the Cardiac Anomaly Collection of McGill Museum.)

Fig. 4.—Diagram showing circulation in tricuspid and pulmonary stenosis with closed septum. The pulmonary artery is here hypoplasic, the right ventricle greatly hypertrophied and the right auricle dilated. (Drawing by P. Larivière.)

Fig. 5.—Heart in tricuspid and pulmonary stenosis of inflammatory origin with pinhole pulmonary orifice surmounted by recent vegetations. Great hypertrophy of right ventricle and auricle.*

(1) The fused pulmonary cusps with raphe *a,a,a*; *b*, central pinhole orifice surmounted by vegetations; (2) conus of right ventricle showing *a*, puckering of myocardium; *b*, thickened endocardium; (3) lower bulbar orifice formed by *a*, crista supraventricularis, *b*, trabecula supramarginalis; (4) interventricular septum.

From a young girl aged 14 with severe dyspnoea and marked cyanosis and

* Specimen in the Cardiac Anomaly Collection of McGill University.

clubbing, healthy and active, until the age of nine, when cyanosis first began following sore throats. Precordial bulging, rough systolic thrill maximum at third left interspace, rough systolic murmur maximum at apex and pulmonary area. R.B.C. 7,600,000, leucocytes 22,000. Died in dyspnoeic attack. (Reported by M. E. Abbott, D. S. Lewis and W. W. Beattie, *Amer. J. Med. Sci.*, 1923, **165**: 636, Case 1. Drawing by W. W. Beattie of Specimen No. 9905 in McGill Museum.)

B

Fig. 6.—Diagram showing the circulation in localized defect of the interventricular septum with dextroposition of the aorta. (From Abbott and Dawson, *Internat. Clin.*, 924, **4**: 170, Fig. 9.)

Fig. 7.—Heart, x-ray and electrocardiogram from a case of interventricular septal defect with dextroposition of aorta and great dilatation of pulmonary artery (Eisenmenger complex). Death from cerebral abscess.

a. View of exterior of heart, showing the great hypertrophy of the right ventricle especially of the conus and great dilatation with hyperplasia of pulmonary artery.

b. Teleoroentgenogram of the heart, showing huge pulmonary arc and right-sided hypertrophy.

c. The left ventricle laid open to show a large interventricular septal defect 2 cm. across with sclerosed border, and the somewhat hypoplasic dextroposed aorta. *A*, right anterior (coronary) aortic cusp; *B*, ventricular septal defect.

d. Electrocardiogram showing right preponderance. Split R and S, and slight delay in conduction (bundle-branch block).

From a young man aged 21 years, with hoarseness and aphonia since age of 13 (from pressure of the huge pulmonary conus on recurrent laryngeal nerve). Slight cyanosis and dyspnoea on exertion but no clubbing. Loud systolic murmur over heart, maximum at pulmonary area and soft diastolic to left of sternum. Cerebral symptoms developed two weeks before death from large abscess in right front parietal region (streptococcus haemolyticus). The septal defect measured 2 cm. across, the pulmonary artery 8 cm. and the aorta 6 cm. in circumference. (From the Medical Clinic of the Clifton Springs Sanatarium, reported by Baumgartner and Abbott, *Amer. J. Med. Sci.*, 1929, **177**: 639.)

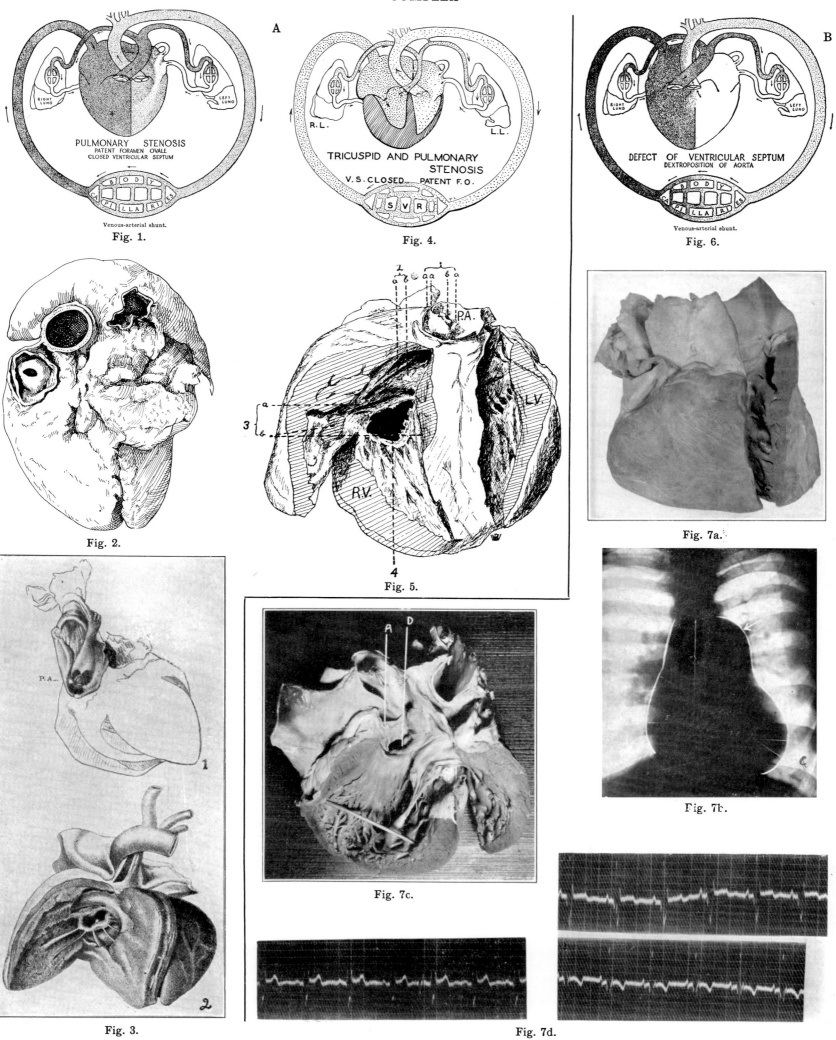

Fig. 1.

PULMONARY STENOSIS
PATENT FORAMEN OVALE
CLOSED VENTRICULAR SEPTUM

Venous-arterial shunt.

Fig. 4.

TRICUSPID AND PULMONARY STENOSIS
V.S. CLOSED   PATENT F.O.

Fig. 6.

DEFECT OF VENTRICULAR SEPTUM
DEXTROPOSITION OF AORTA

Venous-arterial shunt.

Fig. 2.

Fig. 5.

Fig. 7a.

Fig. 3.

Fig. 7c.

Fig. 7b.

Fig. 7d.

PLATE XIX

PULMONARY STENOSIS AND ATRESIA WITH DEFECT OF VENTRICULAR SEPTUM (TETRALOGY OF FALLOT)

The combination presented in this plate of pulmonary stenosis and septal defect with dextroposition of the aorta and hypertrophy of the right ventricle, conveniently known as the "tetralogy of Fallot," is almost invariably present in the developmental form of this lesion and contrasts sharply in most respects with the inflammatory, purely valvular type of pulmonary stenosis (Pl. XVII*A*). In the group under consideration the entire pulmonary tract is usually narrowed and hypoplasic, the pulmonary valve is bicuspid and its leaflets frequently fleshy in character and the conus is narrow and deformed or constricted at its lower bulbar orifice, while the wide thick-walled aorta rides above the large defect in the interventricular septum receiving blood through this from both ventricles. The whole appearance is highly suggestive of the relationships that would result from the uncovering of the right reptilian aorta and obliteration of the left in the delayed torsion of Spitzer's theory (his types I and II of transposition) and is of great interest in this connection.

As Fallot himself pointed out, this is by far the commoner type of pulmonic stenosis, and it was present in 77 per cent of the 110 cases of pulmonary stenosis and in 66 per cent of the 40 cases of atresia classed as the primary lesion in the writer's chart of 1000 cases analyzed (pp. 60–61). It is also the most important from the clinical standpoint, because of the relative frequency with which these patients, despite the high degree of oxygen unsaturation which they invariably present, attain adult life, the maximum age being approximately 25 years and the average in 83 cases being 12¾ years, if we except Lafitte's patient who was 36, and Paul White's musician who reached the unprecedented age of 59 years 9 months. The raised pressure in the right ventricle behind the stenosis sends a large venous-arterial shunt into this dextroposed aorta through the defect, and the effect of this in the circulation is intensified by increased deoxygenation at the periphery due to the obstruction at the pulmonary orifice, Lundsgaard's *D* and alpha factors acting together to raise oxygen unsaturation high above its threshold value. In addition the long standing capillary changes and the effect of the polycythemia and great hypertrophy of the right ventricle that develop as compensatory features combine to produce the most pronounced symptomatology of morbus coeruleus ever seen in adult life, with enormous clubbing of the extremities and a polycythemia varying from 7,000,000 to 12,000,000.

On the subject of congenital cyanosis see the following references: The pathogenesis and symptomatology of congenital cyanosis and calculation of the venous-arterial shunt: F. P. Parkes Weber, and G. Dorner, *Lancet*, Lond., 1911, **1**: 150; D. Christiansen and Haldane, *J. Physiol.*, 1914, **48**: 244; W. C. Stadie, *J. Exp. Med.*, 1919, **30**: 215; J. A. Harrop, *J. Exp. Med.*, 1919, **30**: 241; J. S. Haldane, *Respiration*, 1922, Yale Univ. Press; J. M. Campbell, G. H. Hunt and E. P. Poulton, *J. Path. and Bact.*, 1923, **26**: 234; C. Lundsgaard and D. D. van Slyke, *Medicine*, 1923, **2**: 1; J. Meakins, L. Dautrebande and W. J. Fetter, *Heart*, 1923, **10**: 153; Weiss and Löwbeer, *Wien. Arch. f. inn. Med.*, 1924, **7**: 367; W. Gravinghoff, *Monatschr. f. Kinderheilk.*, 1927, **35**: 237; J. Barcroft, *The Respiratory Function of the Blood*, 1928, London; M. E. Abbott and W. T. Dawson, *Internat. Clin.*, 1924, **4**: 156; M. E. Abbott, *Blumer's Bedside Diag.*, 1928, **2**: 432–458; D. W. Richards, C. B. Riley and Hiscock, *Arch. Int. Med.*, 1931, **47**: 484; H. N. Segall, *Amer. Heart J.*, 1933, **8**: 628; I. Berconsky, *Rev. Sud. Amer. de Med. et Chir.*, 1934, **5**: 193; P. Cossio and I. Berconsky, *Arch. mal. du coeur*, 1935, **28**: 19. The capillary changes: A. Krogh, *The Anatomy and Physiology of Capillaries*, 1922, Yale Univ. Press; E. Wollheim, *Ztschr. f. klin. Med.*, 1928, **108**: 248; W. Redisch and H. Roesler, *Wien. Arch. f. inn. Med.*, 1929, **16**: 463.

Fig. 1.—Diagram of the circulation in pulmonary stenosis with ventricular septal defect and dextroposition of the aorta (tetralogy of Fallot). (From Abbott and Dawson, *Internat. Clin.*, 1924, **4**: 173, Fig. 12.)

Fig. 2.—Pulmonary stenosis with associated defect of the interventricular septum, dextroposition of the aorta and hypertrophy of right ventricle. View of interior of right chambers. The large aorta arises two-thirds from the right and one-third from the left ventricle, receiving the contents of the latter through the large defect (indicated by arrow). The hypoplasic pulmonary has only two cusps and its conus is small with narrow lower orifice. From a girl of 12 with marked cyanosis and clubbing. (Drawing by Fraser B. Gurd from Specimen 873 in the Cardiac Anomaly Collection of McGill University. Reported by M. E. Abbott, *Blumer's Bedside Diag.*, 1928, **2**: 469, Fig. 320.)

Fig. 3.—Heart-signs record from a case of tetralogy of Fallot, showing seat of maximum intensity of prolonged low-pitched systolic murmur with accompanying thrill at second left interspace, with zone of transmission and higher pitched (second) murmur at angle of left scapula. (Diagram supplied by H. N. Segall. Reference under Pl. XIII, Fig. 6.)

Fig. 4.—Illustrations from C. P. Howard's case of the tetralogy of Fallot.
a. The electrocardiogram from this case. Shows normal rhythm rate 75, marked right axis deviation, high *P* wave and slurring and notching of *R* in lead II.
b. View of aortic vestibule of left ventricle showing large septal defect and the dextroposed aorta above this, which receives blood from both chambers. Note the anomalous chordae in the floor of the defect, also fusion and recent endocarditis of the aortic cusps above it.
c. View of conus arteriosus of right ventricle showing marked stenosis of this region and of pulmonary valve with hypoplasia of pulmonary artery and great hypertrophy of myocardium.

From a man aged 23 with marked cyanosis from childhood and extreme clubbing of nose, fingers and toes. Was mentally deficient, conjunctivae congested, breathing labored, red cell count 10,280,000, haemoglobin 146 per cent, pronounced systolic thrill and rough murmur over precordium and in back, not in neck, maximum at second left interspace, pulmonary second sound faint. Blood pressure 110–60. Subject to curious epileptiform

seizures thought to be due to thromboses in capillaries of brain and cerebral anoxaemia and died in one of these accompanied by frothy haemorrhage from the lungs (oedema). Extensive estimations were made of blood gas findings and calculations of the venous shunt were done by I. M. Rabinowitch. (Reported by H. N. Segall, *Amer. Heart J.*, 1933, **8**: 628. Specimen in the Collection of the Montreal General Hospital, art drawing by Hortense Douglas.)

Fig. 5.—Orthodiagram from Roesler's case of tetralogy of Fallot showing coeur en sabôt, enlarged cardiac shadow to left of median line and prominent aortic knob and double apices on left border. The arrows indicate the two apices of the heart seen in this condition, the lower being that of the greatly hypertrophied right ventricle which curves upward from below, and the upper that of the smaller left chamber. (From the article by H. Roesler. *Wien. Arch. f. inn. Med.*, 1928, **15**: 507.)

Fig. 6.—Pulmonary atresia with defect of the interventricular septum and widely patent ductus arteriosus. The defect is guarded on the side of the right ventricle by a false valve anchored to its walls by two anomalous chordae. From a male infant aged 13 days, cyanotic from birth and died in dyspnoeic attack. (From the specimen in the Cardiac Anomaly Collection of McGill University and reported by William Osler, *Montreal Gen. Hosp. Repts.*, 1880, **1**: 186, Case 3.)

Fig. 7.—Roentgenogram in right oblique diameter from a case of pulmonary atresia with ventricular septal defect and dextroposition of aorta (tetralogy). Note the characteristic *coeur en sabôt* effect from the great hypertrophy of the right ventricle. From a cyanotic male infant aged one year. (Reported by M. E. Abbott, *Blumer's Bedside Diag.*, 1928, **2**: 473, Fig. 325.)

Fig. 8.—Diagram of the circulation in pulmonary atresia with aorta from right ventricle and ventricular septal defect. Note the aplasic left chambers and the huge size of the dextroposed aorta. (From Abbott and Dawson, *Internat. Clin.*, 1924, **4**: 174.)

Fig. 9.—Electrocardiogram in tetralogy with high degree partial block. Sinus rhythm with 2:1, 1:1 partial *A–V* block, marked right axis deviation. High *P* waves especially in Lead II; *QRS* slurred in all leads, and deep *Q*3. (Tracing and reading from G. Nicolson.)

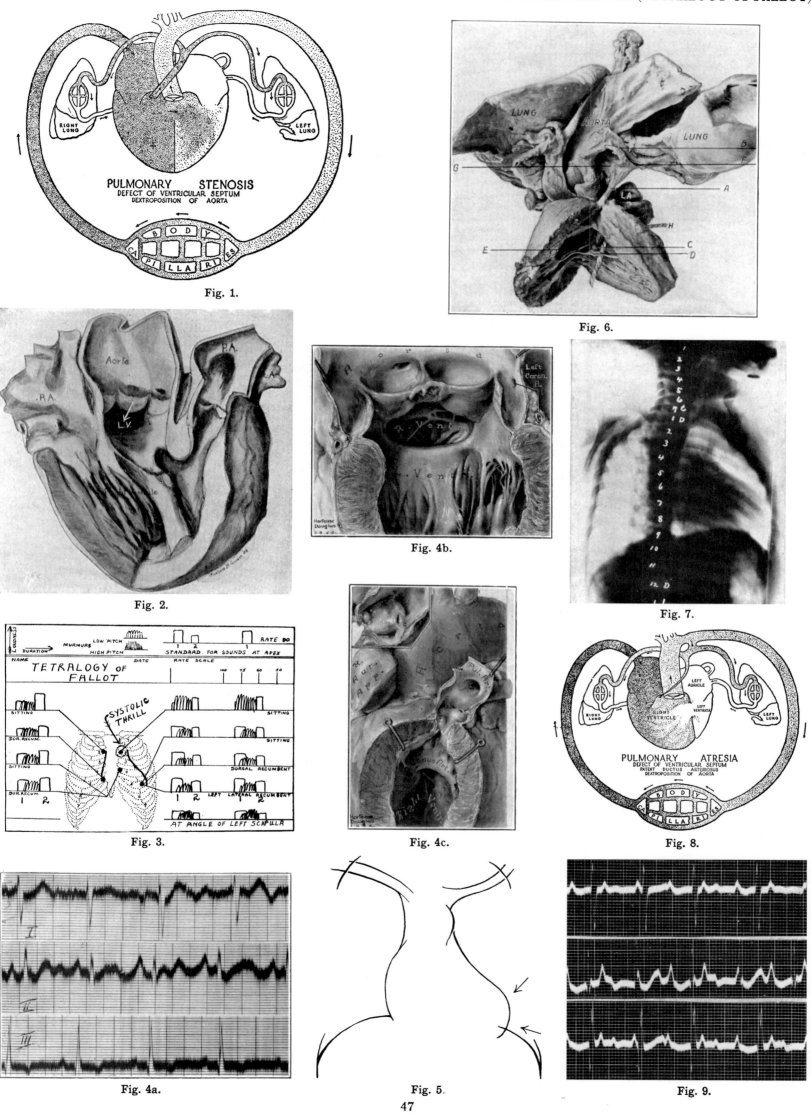

Fig. 1.

Fig. 6.

Fig. 2.

Fig. 4b.

Fig. 7.

Fig. 3.

Fig. 4c.

Fig. 8.

Fig. 4a.

Fig. 5.

Fig. 9.

PLATE XX

PULMONARY ATRESIA WITH CLOSED VENTRICULAR SEPTUM. AORTIC, MITRAL AND TRICUSPID ATRESIA

Pulmonary atresia with closed septum is always, like the less severe grades of pulmonary constriction with this combination (Pl. XVIIIA), of inflammatory origin, due to a valvular endocarditis or, more frequently, to an extensive fibrosis of the myocardium of the underlying conus, setting in in later foetal life after the heart chambers are completely separated. The conditions of the circulation are here much more serious than in the presence of an associated septal defect, for, in the absence of any direct opening into the dextroposed aorta, the venous blood from the right auricle must pursue a circuitous path through the foramen ovale to the left chambers, and thence via the ductus (which is always patent) to the lungs. These are the cases of extreme cyanosis from birth, the true blue baby of morbus coeruleus in whom life is sustained for only a few days or weeks or occasionally months. [A curious exception to this was Costa's case (*Clin. Med. Ital.*, 1930, **61** : 567), of a cyanotic youth with marked clubbing of the extremities who attained his twentieth year, in whom therefore some source of collateral circulation must have existed, else oxygenation could not have been maintained.] These infants usually present a purplish leaden hue of skin with marked dyspnoea and dyspnoeic attacks, and death may take place in one of these or suddenly without apparent cause. The right ventricle is aplasic and the right auricle and left chambers are enormously enlarged while an aorta of great size carries on the entire work of both circulations with the help of the patent ductus and foramen ovale. Such cases were described by Shapiro (*Arch. Path.*, 1930, **9** : 54) and subsequently by Kugel (*l.c.* under Fig. 3*b* below).

The opposite condition of *aortic atresia with closed septum* these authors likewise described as truncus solitarius pulmonalis (shown in Figs. 5, 6 and 9 opposite and in Pl. XXIII, Fig. 4*a*). Here the right chambers are in their turn huge and the large pulmonary artery transmits the blood to the general circulation through the widely patent ductus, while the aorta is reduced at its origin to a blind cord giving off the coronary arteries from its patent distal end and the vessels of the arch higher up, the partly aerated blood reaching these from the pulmonary artery in a retrograde stream through the patent ductus (Fig. 9), while the mitral orifice and left ventricle are aplasic. Cyanosis is extreme and the average duration of life in 12 cases was only four days. Most of these cases are due as in this type of pulmonary atresia to a foetal myocarditis with resultant scarring in the conus wall just below the valves (Pl. XXIII, Fig. 4*b*), as was pointed out by de Zalka (*Frankf. Ztschr. f. Path.*, 1924, **30** : 144).

Mitral and tricuspid atresia are usually of developmental origin, and a septal defect is nearly always associated, producing a special type of cor triloculare. The roentgenogram in tricuspid atresia shows a left-sided enlargement (Fig. 8) that is characteristic and of diagnostic value, as is the left axis deviation seen in the electrocardiogram in these "right-sided lesions" of the cyanotic group. (See on this subject the article by J. Rihl, K. Terplan, and F. Weiss, *Med. Klin.*, 1929.) Mitral atresia is very rare and is usually associated with grave somatic defects. Donnelly's case was, however, a true aplasia (*J.A.M.A.*, 1924, **82** : 1318).

Fig. 1.—Diagram showing course of the circulation in pulmonary atresia with closed ventricular septum, patent foramen ovale and patent ductus. (From Abbott and Dawson, *Internat. Clin.*, 1924, **4** : 181, Fig. 20.)

Fig. 2.—Pulmonary atresia of inflammatory origin. Ventricular septum closed. Ductus arteriosus and foramen ovale widely patent. Left chambers and right auricle dilated and hypertrophied. The large aorta rises in its normal position to the right and posteriorly and the small pulmonary artery passes up on the left to connect with the descending arch through the widely patent ductus (1). The interventricular groove is displaced upward on the right outlining the aplasic right ventricle, the left chamber forming the apex and anterior four-fifths of the heart. (2) The atresic pulmonary orifice.

From a cyanotic infant dying on the ninth day. Case of Edward Bassen, New Haven. (Reported by M. E. Abbott, *Bull. Int. Assn. Med. Mus.*, 1924, **10** : 111.)

Fig. 3.—Congenital atresia of the pulmonary orifice, with closed interventricular septum, absence of tricuspid valve, aplasia and aneurysmal dilatation of right ventricle, patent foramen ovale and ductus arteriosus; truncus aorticus solitarius; single coronary artery.

a. The paraffinized heart showing the huge truncus aorticus and enlarged right auricle with cystic dilatation of right ventricle, bifid apex formed by massive left ventricle, and pulmonary artery forming a solid cord.

b. Roentgenogram showing the huge cardiac shadow of peculiar egg-shaped appearance formed by the dilated right auricle on right above and by the left ventricle on left below.

From an infant cyanotic and dyspnoeic from birth with some clubbing and a rough systolic murmur of peculiar resonant quality, maximum over second left interspace transmitted to apex; dying, aged 6 months, from erysipelas of the vulva. At autopsy there was no trace of the tricuspid valve or its attachments. (From M. A. Kugel, "Two cases of truncus solitarius aorticus (pulmonary atresia)," *Amer. Heart J.*, 1931, **7** : 262.)

Fig. 4.—Diagram showing circulation in aortic and mitral atresia with aplasia of left ventricle, etc. (From Abbott and Dawson, *Internat. Clin.*, 1924, **4** : 182, Fig. 21.)

Fig. 5.—Congenital atresia of aortic orifice from foetal myocarditis, ventricular septum entire, patent foramen ovale, persistent ductus, mitral aplasia, rudimentary left ventricle and auricle. From a baby boy 3 days old, the first of twins. Cyanosis developed on second day and did not decrease on administration of oxygen, no heart murmurs elicited. (Reported by H. R. Wesson and D. C. Beaver, *J. Tech. Meth.*, 1934, **14** : 86, Fig. 2.)

Fig. 6.—Congenital aortic atresia and mitral aplasia with marked concentric hypertrophy of left ventricle and hyperplasia of lining of mural endocardium. Ventricular septum entire, ductus arteriosus widely patent.

a. The ascending aorta and its relationships with the ductus arteriosus and pulmonary trunk. Shows interior of small narrow aorta with occluded aortic valve giving off its branches and emptying through its dilated isthmus into the patent ductus arteriosus which connects it with the descending aorta. (1), anterior view; (2), posterior view.

b. Posterior view of heart showing interior of the small left auricle and aplasic ventricle, in a state of marked concentric hypertrophy, lined by thickened mural endocardium. Apex markedly bifid, formed entirely of right ventricle.

From a male infant, aged 15 days, weighing nine pounds and deeply cyanotic from birth. Cardiac dulness to left axilla and subclavicular region and systolic murmur over upper left chest. Died suddenly. (From Children's Memorial Hospital. Reported by F. W. Wiglesworth, *J. Tech. Meth.*, 1936, **15** : 153. Drawings by P. Larivière, Medical Art Department, McGill University.)

Fig. 7.—Diagram of circulation in tricuspid atresia with defect of interventricular septum. (Drawing by P. Larivière.)

Fig. 8.—Roentgenogram of the thorax, anterior view, in a case of tricuspid atresia. Showing beautifully the typical cardiac shadow in this condition, the enlargement being entirely in the left thorax with absence of pulmonary arc and wide aortic base.

From a cyanotic male infant, aged 6 months, with shortening of right forearm and absence of thumb. Red cells, 6,850,000. Presented a loud systolic murmur, maximum over left base with marked precordial thrill. *Left-axis deviation* with very high PI and PII and deep notching of QRS complex. Diagnosed during life as a three-chambered heart. Tricuspid orifice absent, large persistent ostium primum, small defect of interventricular septum. (From L. M. Blackford and L. D. Hoppe, "Functionally two chambered heart," *Amer. J. Dis. Child.*, 1931, **41** : 1111.)

Fig. 9.—Atresia of ascending aorta which takes origin from coronaries. Pulmonary artery forms descending aorta. Patent ductus arteriosus. Left subclavian below ductus. A female infant aged 4 days, cyanotic at birth, sudden death. (From the Maternity Service of the Royal Victoria Hospital. Reported by M. E. Abbott, *Nelson's Loose-leaf Med.*, 1932, **4** : 297.)

Fig. 10.—Roentgenogram of the case seen in Fig. 6, showing marked cardiac enlargement especially at left upper border.

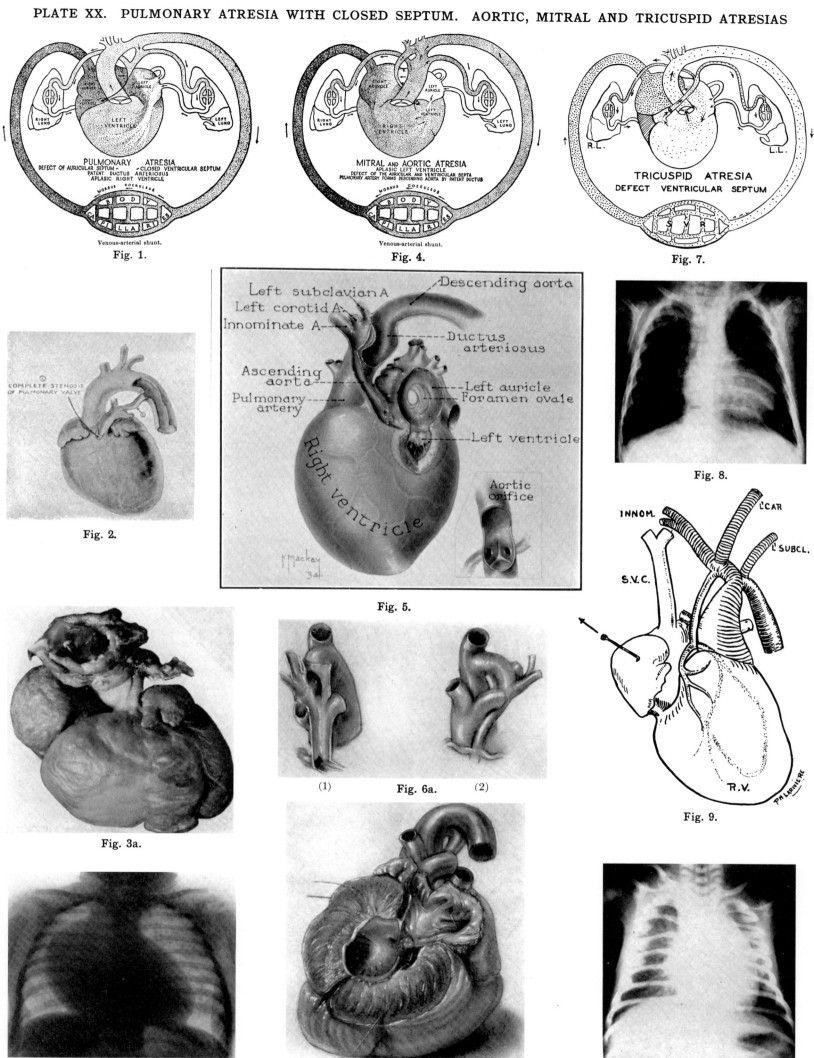

PULMONARY ATRESIA
DEFECT OF AURICULAR SEPTUM — CLOSED VENTRICULAR SEPTUM
PATENT DUCTUS ARTERIOSUS
APLASIC RIGHT VENTRICLE

Venous-arterial shunt.

Fig. 1.

MITRAL and AORTIC ATRESIA
APLASIC LEFT VENTRICLE
DEFECT OF THE AURICULAR AND VENTRICULAR SEPTA
PULMONARY ARTERY FORMS DESCENDING AORTA BY PATENT DUCTUS

Venous-arterial shunt.

Fig. 4.

TRICUSPID ATRESIA
DEFECT VENTRICULAR SEPTUM

Fig. 7.

Fig. 2.

Left subclavian A
Left corotid A
Innominate A
Ascending aorta
Pulmonary artery
Descending aorta
Ductus arteriosus
Left auricle
Foramen ovale
Left ventricle
Right ventricle
Aortic orifice

Fig. 5.

Fig. 8.

Fig. 3a.

(1)   Fig. 6a.   (2)

INNOM.   C CAR
L SUBCL.
S.V.C.
R.V.

Fig. 9.

Fig. 3b.

Fig. 6b.

Fig. 10.

49

PLATE XXI

A. PERSISTENT OSTIUM ATRIO-VENTRICULARE COMMUNE. B. COR TRILOCULARE BIATRIATUM AND BIVENTRICULARE.

A. Combined partial defect of the lower part of the interauricular (persistent ostium primum) and upper part of the interventricular septa, constituting the so-called *persistent ostium atrio-ventriculare commune*, forms a well-recognized group of anomalies, in which a more or less free communication exists between all four chambers of the heart, which functions, where the septal defect is large, as a biloculate organ ("incomplete double heart"). Cleavage of the anterior mitral and deformity of the tricuspid segments is a constant feature of persistent ostium primum and where the interventricular septum is also largely defective a complete separation of each of these cusps into two halves occurs, the contiguous parts of which are continuous each with the other over the free septal border (Fig. 2). Unless the septal defect is very large, cyanosis is absent except as a transient or terminal feature and a loud systolic murmur over the midprecordium and at apex is commonly present. The condition is explained as a failure of upward growth of the ventricular septum combined with an arrest of fusion of the auriculo-ventricular endocardial cushions with the free lower border of the septum primum. A feature of extraordinary interest is the frequent combination of mongolian idiocy with this form of defect and with persistent ostium primum per se (Figs. 2, 3, 4 opposite and Pl. XIV, Fig. 8). This combination calls for explanation.

B. Absence or rudimentary development of one or other of the cardio-vascular septa is the underlying anatomical feature of the group of cases which form the subject of this group and that following (Pl. XXII). In these cases of biloculate and triloculate heart, the main factor in the production of raised oxygen unsaturation is the admixture of venous with arterial blood that takes place in the common chamber (*alpha* shunt). The degree of this venous admixture and the cyanosis that may result therefrom vary, however, according to the location and extent of the defect. Thus in complete absence of the *interauricular septum (cor triloculare biventriculare)* without associated anomalies, little effect will be observed, for the reason that here, just as in localized defects of the auricular septum, the shunt is arterial-venous with possible reversal of flow and the advent of transient or terminal cyanosis. Absence of the interventricular septum (*cor triloculare biatriatum*), on the other hand, leads inevitably to a free admixture of venous with the arterial blood within the common ventricle and to the transmission of this mixed current into the systemic circulation. Cyanosis in these cases is *moderate* in degree in the absence of associated anomalies (*alpha* shunt without *D* factor), the signs of oxygen unsaturation setting in relatively late, with clubbing absent or slight, and the subjects having a fair expectation of life until the third or fourth decade (highest age on record 35 years). In a special group of these cases of great interest (Fig. 9 opposite), an anomalous septum cuts off a small supplementary cavity giving off the transposed aorta (Spitzer's Type IV of transposition). In the Holmes' heart, which is still unique in the literature (Fig. 6), the pulmonary artery arose from this chamber, and the anomalous septum was believed to be the malposed ventricular one (Ngai, *l.c.* below).

(For bibliography on this subject see page 38.)

A

Fig. 1.—**Diagram of the circulation in persistent ostium atrio-ventricular commune.** Note the central opening communicating with all four chambers guarded laterally by single mitral and tricuspid segments. (Drawing by P. Larivière, Medical Art Department, McGill University.)

Fig. 2.—**Persistent ostium atrio-ventriculare commune with completely cleft anterior mitral and septal tricuspid segments, continuous with each other over free border of defective interventricular septum.*** Valvular endo-cardium redundant. Bifid apex. From a female infant, aged 5 months, product of the mother's fourteenth pregnancy, presenting *mongoloid facies* and systolic murmur over whole precordium and terminal cyanosis. Death from bronchopneumonia. (Specimen No. 11353, presented to the writer from the Pathological Service of the New York Hospital by Dr. Robert A. Moore. Drawing by P. Larivière.)

Fig. 3.—**Roentgenograph in left oblique diameter in a case of persistent ostium atrio-ventriculare commune in mongolian idiocy.** Shows great enlargement of the cardiac shadow in the transverse diameter. From a female infant, aged one year, dying of lobular pneumonia. Mongolian facies, flattened nose, bilateral internal strabismus and slant eyes with foetal type of detachment of retina. Heart showing persistent ostium atrio-ventricular commune surrounded by five distinct cusps and no other cardiac anomaly. (Reported by Louise Meeker, *J. Tech. Meth.*, 1935, **14**: 72, Fig. 1.)

Fig. 4.—**Persistent ostium atrio-ventriculare commune in a case of mitral atresia and absence of transverse aortic arch.*** The hypoplasic ascending aorta ends after giving off the innominate and left carotid, and the bicuspid pulmonary artery forms the descending arch through a widely patent ductus. From a cyanotic infant dying at 15 hours, showing stigmata of mongolian idiocy. Mother fifth para, aged 43 years. (From the Maternity Service Division of the Royal Victoria Hospital, Specimen No. 9835, reported by M. E. Abbott, *Nelson's Loose-leaf Med.*, 1932, **4**: 223, Fig. 10.)

B

Fig. 5.—**Circulation in complete absence of the interventricular septum (cor triloculare biatriatum).** (From Abbott and Dawson, *Internat. Clin.*, 1924, **4**: 178, Fig. 18.)

Fig. 6.—**Dr. Holmes' famous case of cor biatriatum triloculare with malposed ventricular septum cutting off a small cavity giving off the pulmonary artery in normal (not transposed) relations.***
a. Anterior view of the heart laid open to show the interior of the large common ventricle and the small supplementary chamber which communicates with the large one by a diamond-shaped defect in a short muscular

rudimentary septum and gives off from its left upper border the pulmonary artery (seen cut across on the opposite side of the picture). The aorta arises posteriorly in the median line. The right auricle is hugely dilated.
b. **Diagrammatic sketch by R. Tait Mackenzie, showing course of the circulation in this case,** the mitral and tricuspid orifices opening into the common ventricle and the small chamber situated above and anteriorly giving off the pulmonary artery in its normal position.
From a young man aged 22 with moderate cyanosis from childhood, increasing on exertion, who suffered from attacks of palpitation, shortness of breath and pain over heart, in one of which he died. (From Specimen No. 14.123[1], reported by Andrew F. Holmes, first Dean of the Medical Faculty of McGill University. *Tr. Edin. Med. Chi. Soc.*, 1824; republished by M. E. Abbott, *Montreal Med. J.*, July, 1901; also in *Osler's Modern Med.*, 1927, **4**: 702; *Nelson's Looseleaf Med.*, 1932, **4**: 278.)

Fig. 7.—**Diagram of the circulation in cor triloculare biventriculare with arterial trunks transposed.** (Drawing by P. Lariviere.)

Fig. 8.—**Cor triloculare biventriculare in a case of isolated mirror-picture dextrocardia** with persistent omphalo-mesenteric bay and displaced right pulmonary veins. a. anterior, b. posterior view.
From a cyanotic infant aged 17 days. Faint prolonged systolic murmur at base to right of sternum, heart greatly enlarged. The pulmonary artery formed the descending aorta through the widely patent ductus. Six supernumerary splenules. (Reported by Bret Ratner, M. E. Abbott and W. W. Beattie, *Amer. J. Dis. Child.*, 1921, **22**: 508.)

Fig. 9.—**Cor biatriatum triloculare with malposed septum cutting off a small separate chamber which gives off the transposed aorta.** The heart laid open to show the interior of the large common ventricle, at the left upper angle of which is seen a short rudimentary septum cutting off the small separate chamber which forms a definite bulb around the base of the large aorta, which vessel arises from it in transposed relations and is coarctated at the isthmus.
The patient was a well-developed boy aged 9 years, who presented no cyanosis except when in swimming and had always been active. There was asymmetry of the left chest with flaring of the lower ribs and precordial bulging and a widely diffused heaving impulse; also a loud systolic murmur maximum at the apex with middiastolic roll and occasional extrasystoles. At autopsy the heart weighed 700 gm., the ventricle was 22 mm. thick, the small chamber 3 cm. deep, and the aorta was 2 cm. in diameter at its origin but narrowed at the left subclavian to 8 mm. Foramen ovale patent, ductus closed. (From an unpublished case in the Children's Service of the Massachusetts General Hospital. Reported to the writer by M. Moriarty Glendy, R. E. Glendy, and P. D. White. Drawing by Muriel McLatchie, Medical Artist of above hospital.)

* Specimen in the Cardiac Anomaly Collection of McGill University.

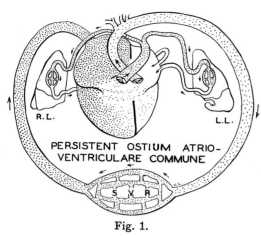

Fig. 1.

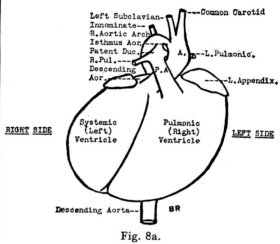

Fig. 5.

Venous-arterial shunt.

Fig. 7.

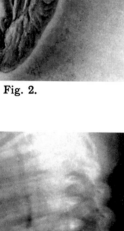

Fig. 2.

Fig. 6a.

rud. cav

Fig. 8a.

Fig. 3.

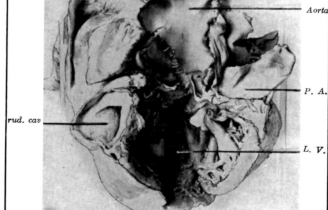

Fig. 8b.

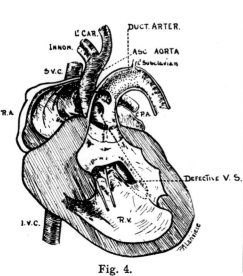

Fig. 4.

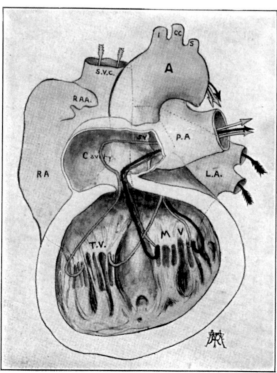

Fig. 6b.

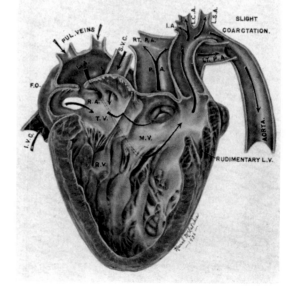

Fig. 9.

PLATE XXII

A. COR BILOCULARE.   B. PERSISTENT TRUNCUS ARTERIOSUS

A. Complete absence of both auricular and ventricular septa, *true cor biloculare*, is a rare condition, usually associated with grave anomalies such as persistent truncus (Fig. 7), displaced pulmonary veins, etc.   As such it constitutes one of the three most extreme forms of morbus coeruleus that exist, the other two being pulmonary atresia and transposition of the great trunks both with closed ventricular septum (Pl. XVIII and XXIII).   Such subjects present profound cyanosis from birth and die in very early infancy.   In some cases, however, when a free collateral circulation or an associated transposition has provided a more favorable path for the circulation, early adult life may be attained.   The highest age on record is that of Rudolf's patient, a cyanotic girl with marked clubbing and dyspnoea who died at 16 of pulmonary tuberculosus; and that of Wood and Williams, a mulatto servant maid presenting the same picture and dying at 15 of purulent meningitis.   In the former case the great trunks were transposed, but in the latter apparently not.

B. Persistent Truncus Arteriosus.   In this interesting condition either the aortic septum is completely absent or the single large arterial trunk that emerges from the base of the right ventricle presents on its interior wall a crescentic ridge indicating its beginning septation (partial truncus, Figs. 3*b* and *c*).   A ventricular septal defect is always associated, and the blood supply to the lungs is derived from larger branches given off from the primitive truncus well above the aortic valve.   In addition a collateral circulation to the limbs is usually developed either from the bronchial or oesophageal arteries or through anomalous vessels from the descending aorta.   As a result these cases fall clinically into the group of marked but not extreme cyanosis, with onset of symptoms frequently delayed until the end of the first year in life and with clubbing as a marked feature.   The average duration in 21 cases was 4 years but the case by Carr, Goodale and Rockwell lived to the age of 36.   A systolic murmur probably generated at the septal defect is usually present.

In the classic type of this condition first described by Preisz, the large anomalous trunk is supplied with four semilunar cusps, and this is theoretically to be expected; for in embryonic life the primitive aorta has four distal bulbar swellings, two of which become subdivided in the descent of the aortic septum, making six valvular segments, three in the aorta and three in the pulmonary artery respectively, so that, in the absence of septation, four valve segments should theoretically persist.   Hulse indeed definitely rejected cases in which there are only three cusps as not being examples of true truncus.   However, a number of well-authenticated cases with only three cusps exist, including the two reported by the writer (Figs. 5 and 6) and in Carr's case the valve was bicuspid.   A very interesting point elicited by recent studies, and illustrated here by the case of Allan Roos (Fig. 8*a*), is the embryonic condition of the fleshy and irregularly thickened aortic cusps.   Rigidly to be excluded from this category of persistent truncus are the cases of pulmonary or aortic atresia reported under the title truncus solitarius aorticus or pulmonalis as the case may be, in which a large trunk functions for both circulations in the place of the obliterated pulmonary artery or aorta, the vestiges of which are traceable as a cord ending blindly at the heart.   Such cases are readily differentiated from true persistent truncus for the entire configuration of the heart is different, and examination usually reveals an aplasic ventricle hidden in the fleshy wall of one or other ventricle behind the atresic orifice (*cf.* Pl. XX, Fig. 9).

A. Cor biloculare: R. D. Rudolf, *Anat. Soc. Great Brit. and Ireland*, 1900, Feb. 17–19; L. Rivet and L. Girard, *Arch. des mal. du coeur*, 1913, **6**: 720; R. H. Wood and G. A. Williams, *Amer. J. Med. Sci.*, 1928, **175**: 242.   *B.* Persistent truncus arteriosus: H. Preisz, *Beitr. path. Anat.*, 1890, **7**: 283; N. W. Ingalls, *Anat. Rec.*, 1915, **10**: 9; W. Hulse, *Virch. Arch.*, 1918, **225**: 16; W. Klemke, *Zbl. Path.*, 1925, **36**: 307; H. M. Zimmerman, *Amer. J. Path.*, 1927, **3**: 617; G. Pezz, and G. Agostoni, *Arch. des mal. du coeur*, 1928, **21**: 18; K. H. Finley, *Amer. J. Path.*, 1930, **6**: 317; P. F. Shapiro, *Arch. Path.*, 1930, **9**· 54, Case I; A. Feller *Virch. Arch.*, 1931, **279**: 869; E. M. Humphreys, *Arch. Path.*, 1932, **14**: 671; D. C. Beaver, *Arch. Path.*, 1933, **15**: 51; F. B. Carr, R. H. Goodale and A. E. P. Rockwell, *Arch. Path.*, 1935, **19**: 833; A. Roos, *Amer. J. Dis. Child.*, 1935, **50**: 966.

A

Fig. 1.—Diagram of the circulation in complete absence of the cardiac septa (cor biloculare) with transposition of the great arterial trunks. (From Abbott and Dawson, *Internat. Clin.*, 1924, **4**: 177, Fig. 15.)

Fig. 1.—Cor biloculare with transposition of arterial trunks, partial situs inversus of viscera and imperforate anus.   From a male infant aged 8½ months.   Mother fourth para, had mental illness in early weeks of pregnancy.   Died of erysipelas following measles and otitis media.   *No cyanosis* throughout.   At autopsy heart very large, common auriculo-ventricular orifice with three cusps between common auricle and ventricle.   Pulmonary artery lies transposed behind aorta, is hypoplasic, without valve.   Stomach, duodenum and pancreas totally, liver caecum and appendix partly transposed.   (Case in the service of E. Weiss.   Reported by M. E. Abbott, *Blumer's Bedside Diag.*, 1928, **2**: 494, Fig. 340.)

B

Fig. 3.—Feller's diagrams showing the essential features in his three cases of persistent truncus.

a. Complete persistence of the primitive truncus.   Both pulmonary arteries arise from it before the origin of great vessels.   No trace of septum in its interior.   Three semilunar cusps, one with raphe behind it.   Large septal defect.   Male, aged one week.

b. Persistent truncus with partial division of interior by sickle-shaped septum.   This incompletely separates a large left anterior chamber giving off the pulmonary arteries from a smaller right posterior one, which represents the ascending aorta and gives off the innominate and left subclavian, and after the narrow isthmus (*ai*), the left subclavian arteries (*ss*).   The truncus is 7.2 cm. wide and rises above a septal defect 2.5 cm. across and is provided with three large semilunar cusps with thickened edges, behind one of which is a raphe separating the two coronary orifices from each other.

c. Common truncus partially divided by curving longitudinal ridge to left of which pulmonary arteries are given off.   Four semilunar cusps numbered to indicate bulbar swellings from which they are derived, small septal defect.   Female aged 2 days.   *S.ap.* septum aortico-pulmonale; *S.ip.*, septum interpulmonale; *ps*, pulmonalis sinistra; *pd*, pulmonalis dextra; *cd*, coronaria dextra; *cs*, coronaria sinistra; *D.A.*, ductus arteriosus.   (From *Virch. Arch.*, 1931, **279**: 869; reproduced in *Nelson's Loose-leaf Med.*, 1932, **4**: 283.)

* Specimen in the Cardiac Anomaly Collection of McGill University.

Fig. 4.—Diagram showing the circulation in persistent truncus arteriosus with defect of interventricular septum (venous-arterial shunt). (From Abbott and Dawson, *Internat. Clin.*, 1924, **4**: 177, Fig. 16.)

Fig. 5.—Persistent truncus supplied with three semilunar cusps giving off main pulmonary arteries and accessory branches (collateral circulation) from ascending part of right aortic arch.   Single right coronary.*   The common trunk is 3.2 cm. wide and arises above a septal defect 1.2 cm. across.   Three anomalous accessory branches pass from the ascending (right) arch to the right lung.   Left innominate artery.   From a cyanotic infant aged 2 months. (Specimen No. 10237 in McGill Medical Museum presented from Childrens' Memorial Hospital.)   *Acc.P.A.*, accessory pulmonary artery.

Fig. 6.—Large common arterial trunk rising from hypertrophied right ventricle above septal defect.   Three semilunar cusps.   Septal defect.*   From a boy aged 5 with cyanosis and clubbing since his third year.   Intelligence above the average, paroxysmal dyspnoea and epileptiform convulsions.   Partial autopsy, aorta cut off too short to determine source of pulmonary blood supply.   (From Specimen No. 1311 presented to McGill Museum by McKenzie Forbes.   Reported by M. E. Abbott, *Osler's Mod. Med.*, 1927, **4**: 708, Fig. 68.)   *A.*, Persistent truncus; *B.*, right auricles; *C.*, defect of ventricular septum; *D.*, muscular column; *E.*, auricular septum.   *H.V.* right ventricle.

Fig. 7.—Diagram showing the circulation in cor biloculare with persistent truncus (intense morbus coeruleus). (From Abbott and Dawson, *Internat. Clin.*, 1924, **4**: 178, Fig. 17.)

Fig. 8.—From a case of persistent truncus with partial division of lumen, right aortic arch, and embryonic thickening of semilunar cusps.

a. Photomicrograph of ostium showing nodular free margin of the valve composed of homogeneous lightly stained myxomatous tissue with notable absence of elastic fibres.   (Weigert's-safranine stain; X 18.)

b. Roentgenogram of heart showing 200 per cent enlargement (W. E. Anspach) and an oval density on right side above (indicated by arrows), probably produced by right aortic knob.

From a female infant with moderate cyanosis of lips and nailbeds and loud systolic murmur over whole precordium, dying at 17 days from acute nutritional disturbance.   (Reported by Allan Roos, *Amer. J. Dis. Child.*, 1935, **50**: 966.)

PLATE XXII. A. COR BILOCULARE. B. PERSISTENT TRUNCUS ARTERIOSUS

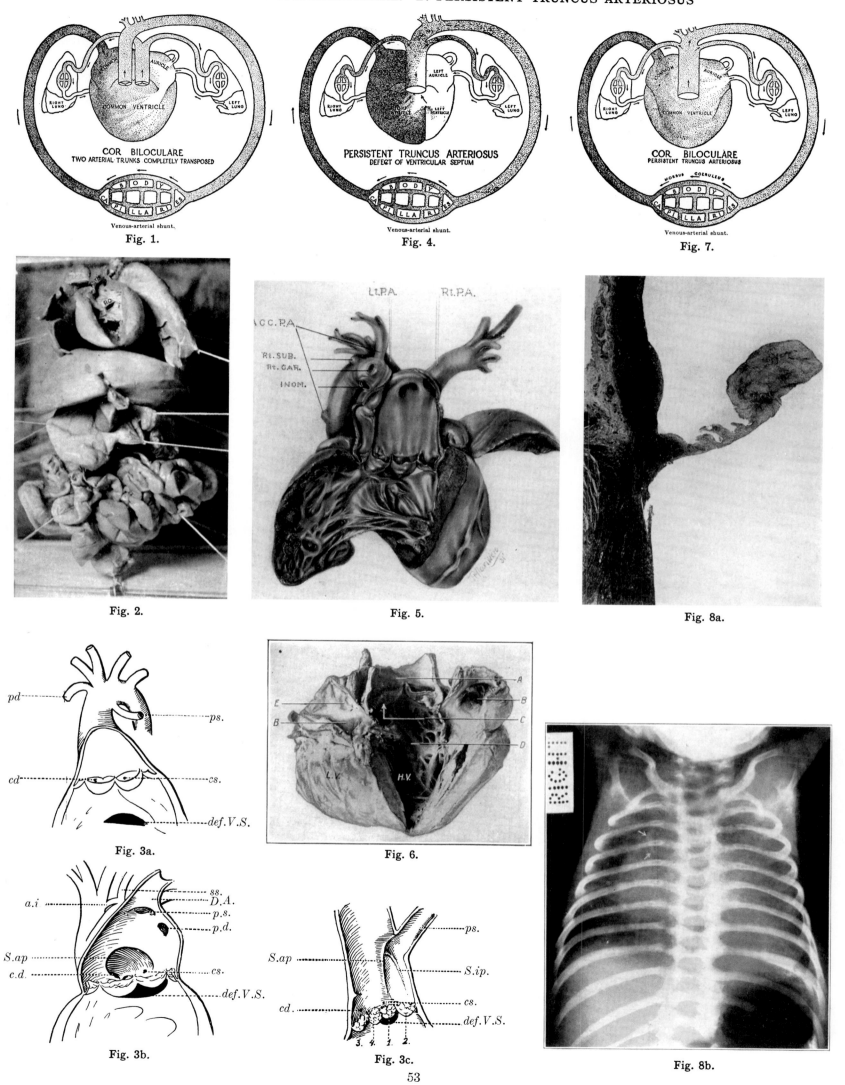

Fig. 1.

Fig. 4.

Fig. 7.

Fig. 2.

Fig. 5.

Fig. 8a.

Fig. 3a.

Fig. 6.

Fig. 3b.

Fig. 3c.

Fig. 8b.

PLATE XXIII

COMPLETE TRANSPOSITION OF GREAT TRUNKS WITH CLOSED VENTRICULAR SEPTUM

Complete or, in Spitzer's terminology, *"crossed" transposition of the great trunks* is a truly extraordinary and quite inexplicable phenomenon, when considered from the purely ontogenetic standpoint. For it must be recognized that this anomaly, in which the aorta arises from the right ventricle and the pulmonary artery from the left in an otherwise normal heart, cannot be the result of a mere arrest of growth, and can be explained only by the operation of additional unknown factors. The only other view possible would be to regard such acondition as a spontaneous aberration, constituting as it does a bewildering contradiction to the fundamental principles underlying the evolution of the cardiac architecture to meet the needs of the double circulation. Thus, in spite of Rokitansky's brilliant morphological contribution to the elucidation of this subject, it was not until it was approached from what may be termed the teleological viewpoint that the enquiry into this intriguing problem yielded any directly fruitful results. The comparative anatomy studies of Keith, Robertson and others (Pl. II and III) first established the phylogenetic basis of these graver cardiac defects and may be said to have pointed the way to further advances. Spitzer's spectacular explanation is in line with these earlier investigations but goes a step farther, harking back to the remote ancestry of the race and the inheritance of suppressed primordial tendencies which the anomaly unveils. Starting from the principle that very early arrest may fix, in the growing embryo, certain rapidly evanescent atavistic traits characteristic of a common ancestral stem, which have since become submerged in the mammalian and specialized in the reptilian orders, this author has developed, with what appears to us to be quite irrefutable logic, his now well recognized and, we believe, generally accepted *detorsion theory*. Briefly stated, this claims that early arrest in the bulbar region of the primitive heart tube inevitably interferes with the clockwise torsion that takes place in this region in normal growth; that any such lack of torsion, (i.e., detorsion) will result in the obliteration of the normal human (left) aorta, and the *persistence of the reptilian right aorta*, which is evanescent in the human embryo but now appears in permanent form as the "transposed" vessel, standing in abnormal relation to the pulmonary artery and other right ventricular structures (Pl. IV); and that this phylogenetic survival of an atavistic structure and its development on an ontogenetic basis are the actual causative factors in this group of grave cardiac anomalies.

Clinical Aspects.—In complete transposition with closed septum, which is the subject of this plate, the conditions of the circulation are the worst conceivable as compatible with life. The venous blood entering the right auricle is transmitted in part through the circuitous route of the patent foramen ovale to the left chambers and thence to the pulmonary artery and in part to the right ventricle whence it passes unaerated through the transposed aorta to the systemic circulation and is returned to the right auricle without aeration by the systemic veins; while the aerated blood returned from the lungs to the left auricle passes straight back to these organs through the pulmonary artery except for a small part which, mixed with venous blood from the right auricle, escapes through the patent ductus to the general circulation. A vicious circle is thus created (Fig. 5) and results in the most extreme form of congenital cyanosis that occurs. Except in the rare cases in which a collateral supply to the lungs develops, these subjects survive only a few days or weeks and present from birth the deep mulberry hue of a true morbus coeruleus. Physical signs when present are generated at the foramen ovale or patent ductus, which latter is, however, occasionally closed (Fig. 3b). The right heart behind the transposed aorta is always greatly hypertrophied and a right preponderance exists. The highest age recorded is **11 years**, average in 31 other cases, 1¾ months.

Acknowledgment is here expressed to Dr. Morris Lev of Chicago for access to his beautiful translation of Spitzer's great monograph (1923).

(For bibliography on this subject see page 38.)

Fig. 1.—Diagram showing the circulation in complete (crossed) transposition of the great arterial trunks with closed ventricular septum. **Morbus coeruleus.** (From Abbott and Dawson, *Internat. Clin.*, 1924, **4**: 179, Fig. 18.)

Fig. 2.—Complete (crossed) transposition of great trunks, aorta from right pulmonary from left ventricle. Ventricular septum entire, foramen ovale and ductus arteriosus widely patent. The heart and lungs of a cyanotic infant dying one hour after birth. The great trunks arise beside each other, the pulmonary to the left of the aorta, and are of about equal size. The right ventricle is the larger of the two and forms the apex. The ductus is widely patent. Heart otherwise normal. (Drawing by Louis Gross in the Cardiac Anomaly Collection of McGill University. Reproduced in Abbott and Dawson, *Internat. Clin.*, 1924, **4**: 180, Pl. IV.)

Fig. 3.—Complete (crossed) transposition of great trunks, aorta and pulmonary artery from reversed ventricles. Ventricular septum entire and ductus arteriosus closed. Foramen ovale patent. Dilatation of aorta and great hypertrophy of right ventricle.

a. The roentgenogram from this case. The shadow is obliquely globular; it shows a mitral configuration. There is a dilatation of the right lower arch extending almost to the right thoracic wall, which indicates a high degree of dilatation of the right auricle. Pulmonary arc not visible. Aortic shadow widened at base.

b. The heart itself. Noteworthy is the huge size of the transposed aorta which arises in the median line and arches over to the left, giving off the great vessels in their normal relations but somewhat twisted back upon themselves to attain the median line; the distinctly smaller pulmonary trunk which hugs the left side of the aorta on a slightly posterior plane; the enormous hypertrophy of the left ventricle which presents a prominent muscular shoulder below the deep auriculo-ventricular groove and forms four-fifths of the anterior surface and entire lower border and apex of the heart; the dilated right auricular appendix; and the position of the smaller left ventricle at the upper left border, as indicated by the position of the interventricular groove.

c. The electrocardiogram from this case. The tracing shows a sinus rhythm with rate of 98 per minute, no conduction delay and marked right axis deviation. The R-T segment is elevated in leads 1 and 2. S_2 is notched. Q_3 is deep, indicating a right ventricular event.

From a colored infant aged **7 months**, the fourth child of a 30-year-old mother with hypertension. Three siblings and a miscarriage preceded this pregnancy. Admitted acutely ill and cyanotic with labored respiration.

Eyelids puffy, lungs showed dullness in both apices. Liver enlarged and tender. Moderate cranio-tabes. Heart was tremendously enlarged to left and right, the sounds forceful. A loud high-pitched, systolic murmur clearest at base in second to third left interspace. No thrill. Pulmonary second sound was decreased. Death soon after admission from bronchopneumonia. At autopsy *the ductus was represented by a ligamentous cord*. No collateral vessels to the lungs were made out, but the inferior vena cava, which was greatly enlarged, received one of the pulmonary veins. The great hypertrophy of the right ventricle that existed was probably the result of this adaptation. (From the Pediatric Service of St. Luke's Hospital, New York. Reported by G. Nicolson for publication in this Atlas.)

Fig. 4.—Complete transposition of arterial trunks with obliteration of aortic orifice below cusps (aortic atresia). Ventricular septum closed. Diffuse myocardial fibrosis and degeneration, syphilitic? Great dilatation and hypertrophy of left ventricle and dilatation of pulmonary artery which forms descending aorta through widely patent ductus, foramen ovale widely patent.

a. The enlarged heart showing the greatly dilated pulmonary artery arising from the left ventricle and forming the descending aorta through the widely patent ductus arteriosus; the base of the aorta laid open to show three rudimentary cusps above the closed conus orifice, the huge left and aplasic right ventricle. *a*, right auricle; *b*, coronary orifice; *c*, aortic valve; *d*, descending aorta; *e*, left appendix; *f*, mitral valve.

b. Microphotograph of the section taken from the myocardium of the conus of the right ventricle just below the aortic cusps, showing perivascular cell infiltration and extensive fibrosis which evidently caused occlusion of the orifice.

From a deeply cyanotic male infant aged **7 days** with a supernumerary finger on right hand. (Case of Berta Meine, Woman's Hospital of Philadelphia. Reported by Abbott and Dawson, *Internat. Clin.*, 1924, **4**: Fig. V. Drawing of heart by Louise Brecht, Woman's Medical College of Pennsylvania.)

Fig. 5.—Circulation of the blood in transposition of the arterial trunks. The dark colored portion represents the venous blood, which is seen filling the entire systemic circulation, while the arterialized blood (uncolored) is confined to the lesser circulation. Communication through one or other of the foetal passages would be necessary for life. *C.S.*, Cor sinistra; *C.D.*, cor dextra; *P.*, pulmonary artery; *A.*, aorta; *C.S.*, superior cava; *C.J.*, inferior cava; *V.P.*, pulmonary veins. (Adapted from Bokay, *Arch. f. Kinderheilk.*, 1911, **55**: 333; Republished by permission of Lea & Febiger from *Osler's Mod. Med.*, 1927, **4**: 719.)

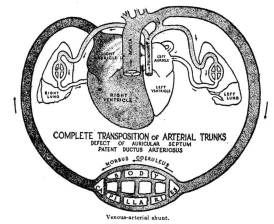

Fig. 1.

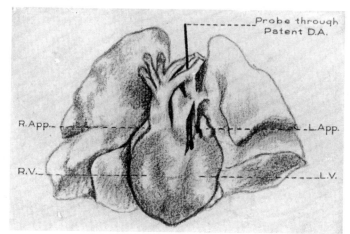

Fig. 2.

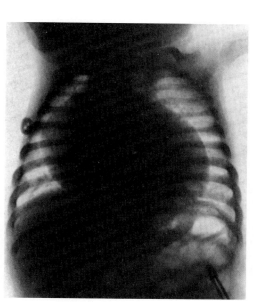

Fig. 3a.

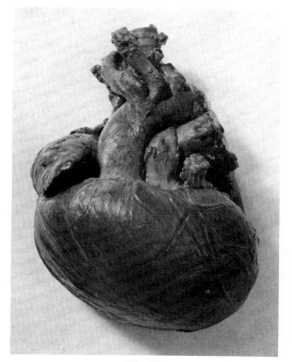

Fig. 3b.

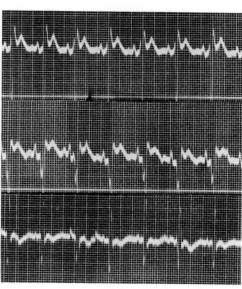

Fig. 3c.

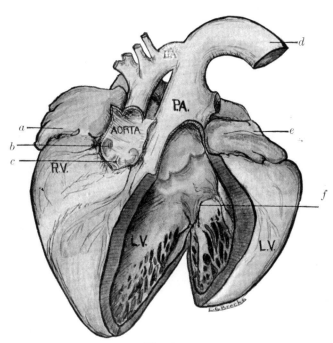

Fig. 4a.

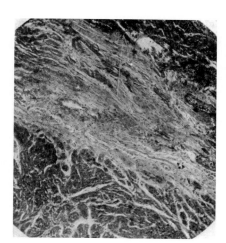

Fig. 4b.

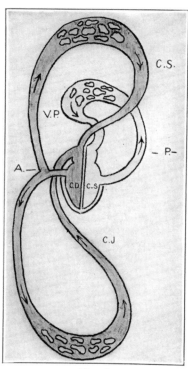

Fig. 5.

55

PLATE XXIV

COMPLETE TRANSPOSITION OF GREAT TRUNKS WITH DEFECT OF INTERVENTRICULAR SEPTUM

As indicated above, complete transposition, where the ventricular septum is entire (Pl. XXIII), is a condition of extreme gravity, only a small fraction of aerated blood reaching the systemic circulation and the unfortunate subjects dying in early infancy. An associated ventricular septal defect, on the other hand, provides distinctly improved circulatory conditions, in that a part of the venous blood from the right auricle passes directly through the defect into the transposed pulmonary artery and thence to the lungs for aeration; and a part of the oxygenated blood returned from the left auricle is transmitted an instant later through the same pathway into the transposed aorta and thence, mixed with unaerated blood from the right auricle, is distributed to the systemic circulation by the same shuttle-like action as is carried on to perfection in the heart of the turtle, with the help of its specially developed auriculo-ventricular valves. Such patients accordingly may live into childhood or early adult life with fairly good cardiac efficiency and only moderate cyanosis. The larger the septal defect the more easily can this circulatory arrangement be carried on, and when other anomalies having a like compensatory effect are associated, life may be sustained with fairly good cardiac efficiency until late middle life.

In the two remarkable cases figured opposite, the auricular septum was completely closed (as in the heart of the turtle) and the ventricular septum was rudimentary, a virtual cor triloculare biatriatum existing; and both were subjects of associated anomalies of a very unusual kind illustrating the remarkable adaptations that may develop in early embryonic life for the maintenance of the circulation. In Case 1 (Figs. 2a and b) the existence of such a grave cardiac anomaly in the host of an omphalositic monster is in itself a very rare occurrence, the autosite being almost always a normal well-developed child; of interest also are the anatomical relations of the mitral and tricuspid segments to the arterial ostia whereby the blood has been propelled into the transposed aorta and pulmonary artery by the shuttle action above described; and the enormous dilatation of the pulmonary circulation that has developed in response to the double demand that existed for oxygenation of the tissue of the parasitic twin.

Case 2 (Figs. 3a, b, 4, 5 and 6) presents a remarkable combination of grave cardiac anomalies unique in our experience in the literature. Space does not permit here the detailed description of this, but the beautiful drawings and diagrams opposite tell their own story. The primary anomaly here was undoubtedly a detorsion defect that apparently involved the auricular as well as the bulbar (ventricular) end of the cardiac tube, so that, in addition to the "crossed" transposition of the great trunks, there existed a *dextroposition of the left auricle behind the right*. Both these chambers have thus come to lie to the right of the great vessels, and the *auricular septum*, which is a strong muscular partition (b in Fig. 3b) completely separating the two auricles, is *malposed*, and lies on a plane anterior and to the right of the rudimentary interventricular septum, with which it is not in continuity, thus explaining the complete heart block that existed. (The writer is deeply indebted to Dr. C. F. Moffatt of the Royal Victoria Hospital, in whose care this patient was during life, for permission to present here the pictorial reproductions of this hitherto unpublished case, to Dr. W. W. Eakin for assistance in studying the clinical laboratory data, and to Miss Harriet Blackstock for the remarkably informing drawings shown.)

This case is possibly analogous to those of *sinistro-position* of the auricles published by O. Wenner, *Virch. Arch.*, 1909, **196**: 127; A. Birmingham, *J. Anat. and Physiol.*, 1892–93, **26**: 139; and S. K. Ngai, *Amer. J. Path.*, 1935, **11**: 309.

Fig. 1.—**Diagram of the circulation in transposition of the great trunks with defect of the interventricular septum and patent ductus.** (From Abbott and Dawson, *Internat. Clin.*, 1924, **4**: 175, Fig. 14.)

Fig. 2.—**Cardiac anomaly in host (complete transposition with rudimentary interventricular septum) in a case of thoracopagus (dipygus) parasiticus.**

a. **The body of a well developed female infant with the lower half of an acardiac parasitic female twin attached at its umbilicus and left thoracic border.** Two small arterioles enter this from the host and constitute its sole blood supply.

b. **The heart and lungs of the host (external view).** The aorta rises on the left anteriorly in the position normally occupied by the pulmonary artery, which emerges behind on the right from the left ventricle and is greatly dilated. The heart is a strong muscular organ, the hypertrophy being chiefly of the right ventricular part. The lungs are voluminous.

From a moderately cyanotic child aged 14 months of good intelligence. No clubbing, palpable thrill felt and unclassified murmur heard all over whole precordium. Died of bronchopneumonia. The ductus arteriosus was widely patent and the pulmonary artery and its terminal branches in the lungs were widely dilated with large thin-walled venous sinuses. (From the Pathological Service of the Hoagland Laboratory, Brooklyn, N. Y. Reported by W. F. Watton and M. E. Abbott, *J. Tech. Meth.*, 1922, **8**: 165.)

Fig. 3.—**Complete (crossed) transposition of great trunks with rudimentary interventricular septum and dextroposed left auricle with malposed auricular septum and complete congenital heart block. Stenosis of conus of right ventricle with hypoplasia of transposed aorta and bulbar septal defect. Supplementary right superior cava from left auricle, and secondary (double) mitral orifice. Patent ductus arteriosus. Dilatation and atheroma of pulmonary artery and veins and arterio-venous aneurysm of lungs (congenital?).**

a. **Interior of aortic vestibule of this case giving off the transposed and greatly dilated pulmonary artery.** Only two of the three pulmonary cusps are visible and a short distance below these are seen the anomalous chordae attached to the double mitral orifice in the anterior segment of the mitral valve. 1, the pulmonary artery; 2, dilated arterioles; 3, rudimentary ventricular septum; 4, double mitral orifice; 5, anomalous chordae.

b. **The heart laid open to show the chambers of both auricles and the sinus of the right ventricle.** The auricular septum has been divided to expose the interior of the large left auricle, which lies directly behind the smaller right auricle. It receives three greatly enlarged pulmonary veins (c) and the supplementary right superior cava in its roof. It is closed below by a competent mitral valve, the anterior segment of which is widely cleft and is the seat of

the double mitral orifice, through which the aerated blood was directed across the aortic vestibule and through the bulbar septal defect into the transposed aorta. The rounded free muscular border of the rudimentary ventricular septum is visible just beneath this cleft segment, and the space above it is crossed by the anomalous chordae of the double orifice. The hugely dilated atheromatous pulmonary artery (P) is seen above the heart in the median line, and below it the large right pulmonary vein (c). S., right superior cava entering right auricle; C., carotid artery; a.-a., the hypertrophied right auricular appendix cut across; b, the divided auricular septum.

Male, aged 20 years, cyanosis and dyspnoea from childhood with cough on exertion and frequent throbbing headaches, marked clubbing with curvature of nails. R.B.C. 7,200,000. Definite precordial bulging and visible pulsation in fourth and fifth left interspaces, questionable systolic thrill over base. Cardiac area enlarged to right and left and above. Soft systolic murmur in third left interspace, pulmonary accentuation, pulse 38, complete heart block. Was able to do very light work, had a slight haemoptysis and a week later died following a sudden terrific pulmonary haemorrhage. (Drawings by H. Blackstock, Medical Art Department, McGill University. From Specimen No. 9839 in the Cardiac Anomaly Collection.)

Fig. 4.—**Roentgenogram from this case** shows enlargement of the cardiac shadow on both right and left sides, enlarged pulmonary arc and marked widening with pulsation of the shadows at the hilum of both lungs. (From the monograph by M. E. Abbott, *Blumers Bedside Diag.*, 1928, **2**: 464, Fig. 316.)

Fig. 5.—**Diagrammatic presentation of the anterior aspect of the heart and great vessels in this case, with insets showing interior of the conus at different antero-posterior levels.** 1, the bulbar septal defect; 2, free border of the rudimentary interventricular septum; 3, the small communication with triple opening between the conus cavity and the sinus of the right ventricle; 4, muscular pillar; A, the hypoplasic aortic arch with patent ductus communicating with the greatly dilated pulmonary artery; SVC, superior vena cava leading into right auricle; a, supplementary right superior cava from left auricle; R.P.A., right pulmonary artery; R.P.V. and L.P.V., dilated right and left pulmonary veins; I.V.C., inferior vena cava. (Drawing by H. Blackstock.)

Fig. 6.—**Electrocardiogram from this case,** showing complete congenital heart block, right ventricular preponderance and inverted T in lead 1. (From *Blumer's Bedside Diag., l.c.* above, Fig. 317.)

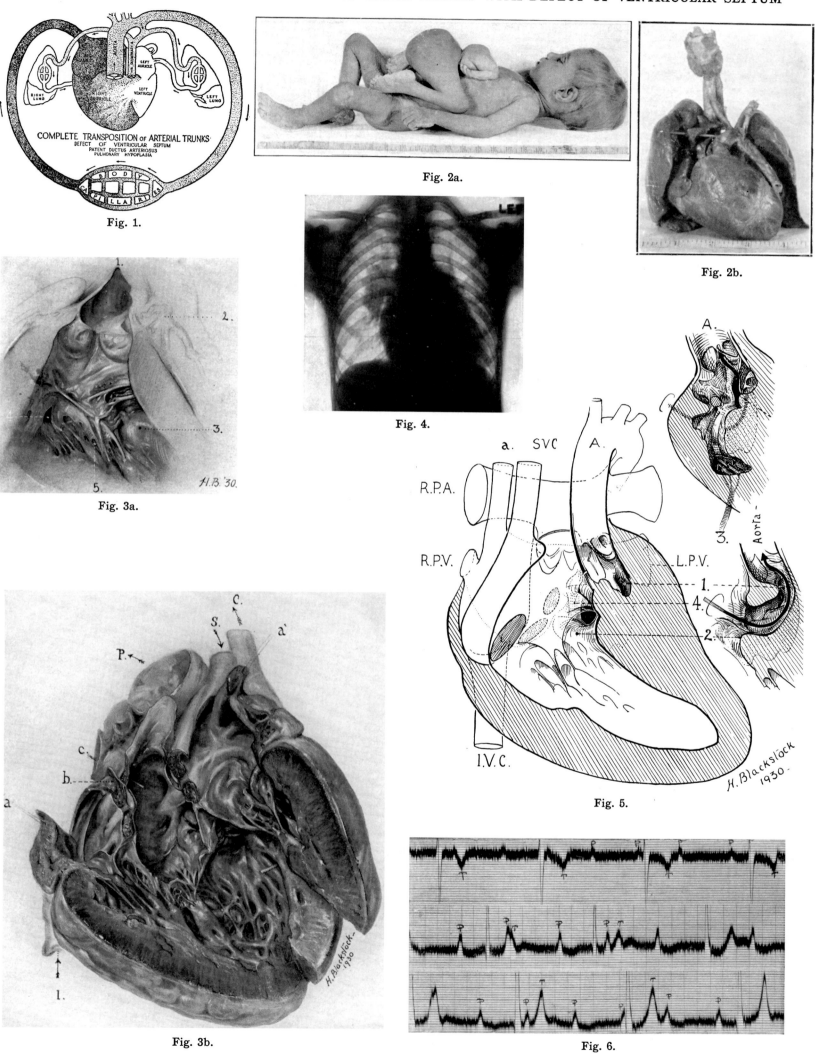

Fig. 1.

Fig. 2a.

Fig. 2b.

Fig. 3a.

Fig. 4.

Fig. 5.

Fig. 3b.

Fig. 6.

57

PLATE XXV

A. DEXTROCARDIA. B. CORRECTED TRANSPOSITION WITH COMPLETE CONGENITAL HEART BLOCK

A. Dextrocardia as a part of a complete situs inversus of the viscera is not, functionally speaking, an anomalous condition, for the path of the circulation is merely reversed without any interference with its physiological course.   Such cases are therefore of no clinical significance and do not come under consideration here.   Mirror-picture dextrocardia with *partial* situs inversus of the viscera, on the other hand, is practically invariably associated with grave cardiac anomalies, which place the cases in the cyanotic group (Figs. 1b, 2a, b, c and 3a and b opposite).   The same applies to "pure" or "isolated" dextrocardia in which there is no situs inversus of the viscera, but in which there is either (a) complete or (b) partial inversion of the heart chambers, or (c) in which there is *no* inversion of the heart chambers but the heart lies to the right of the median line with apex formed by the right ventricle, a condition due to early arrest (not figured here).   This subject is fully reviewed and the above variations classified by H. Roesler with extensive bibliography.   In the case shown opposite of mirror-picture dextrocardia with partial situs inversus of the viscera the absence of right preponderance shown in the electrocardiogram (Fig. 1c) is characteristic of cases complicated by grave cardiac anomalies.

B. "Corrected" transposition is a rare and still incompletely understood phenomenon.   Spitzer acknowledges he has never seen an example, and though Rokitansky's brilliant hypothesis covered eight possible variations, only two of these had been observed by him.   In this phenomenon a complete or crossed transposition has occurred, in that the great trunks arise in reversed relations, but the condition is "corrected" from the functional standpoint in that each trunk is placed in its proper ventricle.   The generally accepted explanation at the present day is that the transposition of the great trunks has been combined with a reversal of the bulbo-ventricular bend with inversion of the ventricles, but this does not seem to explain entirely the facts in the light of Spitzer's detorsion theory.   We owe the privilege of presenting the exquisite example of this unusual anomaly (Fig. 4b) to the courtesy of Dr. Allan Roos of New York, who submitted the specimen to the writer for verification, and the beautiful illustration is the work of Mrs. A. C. Cheney of the Medical Art Department of McGill University.   In it we have an example *par excellence* of this condition in that the aorta arises to the left and anteriorly from the functionally systemic tricuspid valve ventricle here placed on the left side, and the dilated pulmonary artery from the functionally pulmonic mitral valve ventricle which here occupies the right side of the heart.

Complete Congenital Heart Block.—This phenomenon, which was a special feature of the symptomatology of the above case, was apparently explained here by the anomalous relation of the interventricular to the auricular septum, but investigations on this point are being carried out by Dr. Roos.   It was present also in the remarkable case shown in Pl. XXIII, Fig. 3b, and is commonly associated, as was shown by Mönckeberg, with defects of the interventricular septum.

(For bibliography on the above subjects see page 38.)

Fig. 1.—**Mirror picture dextrocardia in partial situs inversus complicated by mitral aplasia.**

a. **Roentgenogram of the heart in this case,** showing the apical portion of the large *coeur-en-sabôt* in the right thorax and the huge "right" auricle forming the left border of the cardiac shadow extending to the left midclavicular line.

b. **Anterior view of heart laid open to show interior of the "right" chambers,** showing the dextroposed aorta arising in the median line and the huge "right" auricle left side receiving the inferior and superior cavae and the displaced left pulmonary veins.   a, tricuspid orifice; b, orifice of coronary sinus; c, orifice of inferior cava.

c. **Electrocardiogram from this case** shows inversion of P and T waves, no preponderance and the leads known as III and II under normal conditions, here replacing one another as leads II and III (characteristic of situs inversus).

A well-developed baby girl aged 14 months with cyanosis from birth and clubbing of fingers and toes.   Apex on the right side, a systolic murmur over base of heart.   Died suddenly just after admission.   The bicuspid and hypoplasic pulmonary artery arose transposed from the systemic ventricle, the mitral valve and ventricle were aplasic, "right" auricle enormously dilated.   (From a case in the service of Graham Ross, Royal Victoria Hospital.   Reported by M. E. Abbott and W. Moffatt, *Canad. Med. Assn. J.,* 1929, **20**: 611.)

Fig. 2.—**Mirror-picture dextrocardia in situs inversus viscerum with multiple associated anomalies (cor biventriculare biatriatum, displaced left pulmonary veins, persistent left superior cava into coronary sinus).**

a. **The left lung and the heart pulled over from behind and laid open to show interior of transposed "right" chambers.**   The right auricle (R.A.) is hugely dilated and receives the superior and inferior cavae on its roof and floor, and the two left pulmonary veins (L.P.V.) on its middle left border and the large coronary sinus on the right below.   It is incompletely separated from the small left auricle (L.A.), which receives the right pulmonary veins (R.P.V.) by a defective auricular septum which presents a widely patent foramen ovale (F.O.) above and the persistent ostium primum below.   The "right" ventricle is hypertrophied and the tricuspid valve surmounted by endocardial excrescences.

b. **Heart everted to reveal interior of the dilated coronary sinus.**   This receives in its roof the persistent superior vena cava and has at its lower border its large crescentic orifice into the "right" auricle.

c. **The thoracic and abdominal viscera of this case in situ,** showing complete transposition.   Liver and appendix on left side, stomach on right, heart in median line with apex in left thorax, dilated "right" auricle receiving pulmonary veins on left and large persistent superior cava entering coronary sinus on right of picture.

From a male infant aged 9 weeks, dying from volvulus of intestines, cyanosis marked on crying, systolic thrill, loud murmur all over precordium.   Ductus patent, no pulmonary stenosis.   (From an unpublished case in the service of Louis Gross, Mount Sinai Hospital, New York.   Drawings by A. C. Cheney from specimen No. 11353 in the Cardiac Anomaly Collection, McGill University.)

Fig. 3.—**Cor biloculare and pulmonary atresia in mirror-picture dextrocardia with partial inversus of viscera.**

a. **Roentgenogram of this case,** showing the large globular cardiac shadow reaching to right axillary border and single arterial trunk.

b. **Semidiagrammatic sketch of the biloculate heart** giving off the large truncus aorticus solitarius from its left upper angle and the atresic pulmonary artery behind and to right of this, communicating with the aortic arch by the patent ductus arteriosus (P.D.A.).   The single auriculo-ventricular orifice is guarded by a common valve with four cusps (A-V.V.) leading into the ventricle from a single auricle, which lies on the left above and receives a common pulmonary vein draining both lungs.

A male infant aged 4 months, "blue" from birth and markedly dyspnoeic, finger nails curved, died just after admission.   Anomalous rotation of pancreas and duodenum, situs inversus of oesophagus and stomach, absence of spleen.   (Reported by M. A. Kugel, *Amer. Heart J.,* 1932, **8**: 280.)

Fig. 4.—**Corrected transposition of great trunks.   Hypoplasia and slight coarctation of aorta.   Anomalous insertion of anterior mitral segment in floor of right auricle and complete congenital heart block.**

a. **The roentgenograph from this case.**   Shows great enlargement of cardiac shadow on left reaching to axillary border.   Enlarged pulmonary arc.

b. **Anterior view of the lungs and heart, the latter laid open to expose interior of both ventricles and the lumina of the great trunks.**   The greatly dilated pulmonary artery (P.A.) arises on the right and somewhat posteriorly from the mitral valve ventricle which occupies the right side of the heart but has the anatomical structure of the normal left chamber and receives venous blood from the right auricle.   The aorta arises to the left and anteriorly from the tricuspid valve ventricle which lies on the left side and receives the aerated blood from the left auricle.

c. **Electrocardiogram from this case showing complete heart block.**   The auricles are beating at a regular rate of 150 per minute.   The ventricular complexes bear no relation to the auricular ones.   In lead I and the first complex seen in lead II, they are of the infraventricular type with a rate of 58 per minute.   Following this the ventricular rate falls to 38 and the complexes are of nodal type.

From a well developed female infant aged 8½ months.   Occasional short periods of transient cyanosis, no polycythemia.   Bradycardia.   Died suddenly.   Liver greatly enlarged, mural endocardium thickened, one pulmonary cusp very small, pulmonary artery 4.5 cm. in circumference, aorta 3 cm., wall fused with pulmonary artery.   (Unpublished case communicated by Allan Roos for publication in this Atlas.   Drawing by A. C. Cheney.)

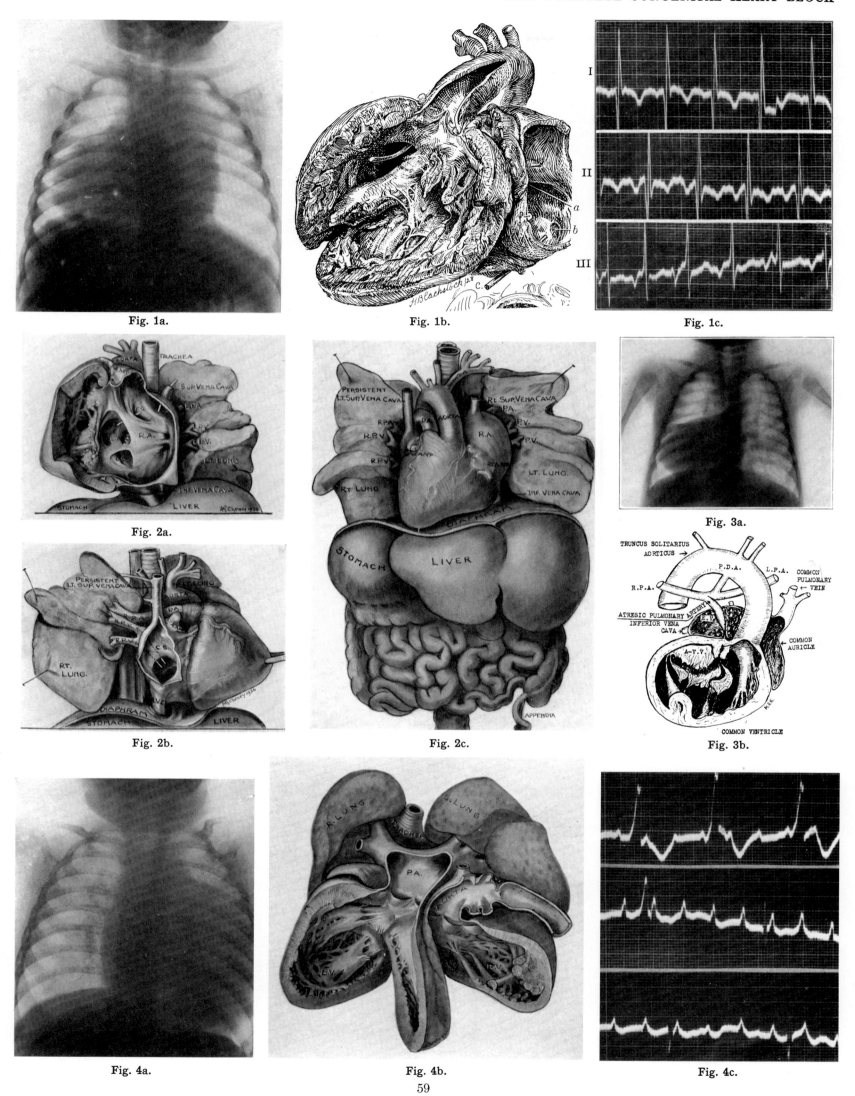

Fig. 1a.

Fig. 1b.

Fig. 1c.

Fig. 2a.

Fig. 2b.

Fig. 2c.

Fig. 3a.

Fig. 3b.

Fig. 4a.

Fig. 4b.

Fig. 4c.

Chart I.—Statistics of Congenital Cardiac Disease (1,000 Cases Analyzed)

Series numbers	Classification of Defects	Number of cases analyzed	Age: Maximum	Age: Minimum	Age: Mean	Sex: Male	Sex: Female	Postmortem: Fetal passages: Patent D. A.	Defect A. S.	Defect V. S.	P.A.: Dilatation	P.A.: Hypoplasia	Aorta: Dilatation	Aorta: Hypoplasia	Dextroposition of aorta	Collateral circulation	Art. dis.: Infective arteritis	Atherosclerosis	Acq. valv. dis.: Acute endocarditis	Chronic lesion	Hypertrophy of heart: R. auricle	R. ventricle	L. auricle	L. ventricle	Assoc. anomal.: In heart	In vessels	Elsewhere	Complications: Paradoxical Embolism	Cerebral Abscess
I	**Anomalies of pericardium:**																												
	1. Pericardial defects.	30	75	Fetus	45	19	6											1			5	4	5	6	3		4		
	2. Diverticulum.	6	52	Adult	45	2	3											2		3	2	2	2	2					
II	**Displacements of the heart:**																												
	1. Ectopia cordis.	7	15m	Fetus	1m	3	3	1	2					1	1						1	2			3	3	4		
	2. "Isolated" Dextrocardia																												
	(a) Without inversion chambers	8	49	Birth	11	3	4	2	5	7		6	4	1	5					2	1	4	1	5	8	5	3	1	
	(b) With inversion chambers.	10	33	Birth	6	7	2	7	7	7	1	7	6		6			1	1		4	5	1	2	10	9	4		
	3. Dextrocardia with situs inversus.	11	58	Fetus	8	3	4	4	8	8		6	4	1	3	1			1	1	1	1	3	4	10	9	11		
	4. Incomplete heterotaxy.	5	6½	6w	1¾	4	1	3	4	3		3	1		3						2	4	4	1	5	4	5		
	5. Dextroposition cordis.	3	41	2½m	26	3										1				1		1			1	1	3		
III	**Anomalies of the heart as a whole:**																												
	1. Bifid apex.	4	40	8	24½		2																				1		
	2. Diverticulum.	3	1½m	Fetus	16d	1	2		1				1												1		2		
	3. Primary congenital hypertrophy.	15	4	Birth	10m	6	4		3		2	1	1	1							8	11	6	13	3	2	2		
	4. Congenital rhabdomyoma.	17	20	Birth	18½	11	3		3	1								1			3	4	1	3	2		10		
	5. Congenital heart block.	3	20	18d	7	2	1	3	1	3	1	1	1	1				1			2	2	2	1	3	3	2		
IV	**Anomalous septa or chordæ:**																												
	1. Anomalous septa (a) in L. A.	10	48	Birth	20	4	6	2	5		3			2				1	1	1	4	9	6	2	3	6	1		
	(b) in R. A.	4	33	16	17½	1	2		2		1			1				1	2	2	1	1	2	1	1				
	(c) in ventricles.	3	39	10w	14	1	2	1	3	3	1	2	2	1	2						1	2		2	3	3			
	2. Anomalous chordæ (a) in L. A.	7	84	35	52	2	2		3									3	1	1	1	1		1	4	1	1		
	(b) in R. A.	5	69	24	46	4	1													1	1	1	1	1	3				
	(c) in ventricles.	6	69	23	36	4	1													4	1	2	1	3					
	(d) in aorta.	5	76	2w	39	3	2						2					2	1	2	1	1	1	1		1	1		
V	**Defects of interauricular septum:**																												
	1. Patent foramen ovale.	40	70	3m	29	15	24		40		15		1	12				6	3	14	28	29	13	10	11	5	8	6	
	2. Defects auricular septum above.	10	64	6m	34	4	5		10		4		2	1				3		4	9	7	4	4	4	7			
	3. Defects auricular septum below.	18	46	8m	19	8	8	1	18		11		1	9					5	8	12	13	12	5	10	1	5		
	4. Multiple defects, auricular septum.	5	52	16	38	3	2		5											1	2	3	2	2	2				
	5. Premature closure F. O.	3	32h	Fetus	18h	2		3	1		3			2							2	3			2	3	1		
VI	**Defects of interventricular septum:**																												
	1. At base (a) without dextroposition.	50	49	Fetus	14½	21	26	2	13	50	16		3	5			8	3	21	14	13	26	10	23	22	4	7	1	
	2. Defects elsewhere or multiple.	5	79	4m	23	2	2	1		1	2			2	1			1		1			1	1		1			
	3. Aneurysms of pars membranacea.	7	60	24	42	6	1		1		1							2			1	1	2	3	2	1	2		
VII	**Complete defects of cardiac septa:**																												
	1. Cor triloculare biventriculare.	5	31	17d	6	2	2	3	4		1	2	1							1	2	2	1		5	2	3		
	2. Cor triloculare biatriatum.	13	35	Birth	7¾	7	3	2	5	13	5	2	3	4	4		1		1	2	4	1	4		10	7	1		
	3. Cor biloculare.	9	16	78h	3¼	3	3	2	9	9	1	3	3	1	7					1	2	2	1	1	9	8	2		
	4. Incomplete double heart.	10	4¾	2m	1½	5	2	4	10	10	4	3	1	4	1			1	1	1	4	4	3	3	8	2	5		
VIII	**Defects of aortic septum:**																												
	1. Persistent truncus (complete defect).	21	25	Birth	4	11	7	1	10	21					19	14		1	2	2	10	15	1	11	13	12	5		
	2. Communication between A. and P. A.	10	48	6d	14	6	3	1	2	1	2		4	1				2	1	1	1	5	1	4	2	4	2		1
	3. Congen. aneur. of right aortic sinus.	12	53	1½	28	11	1			6	4	1	3	2				1	3	4	3	10	4	6	7	2	1		
IX	**Transposition of arterial trunks:**																												
	1. Dextroposition of aorta.																												
	(a) A. from L. V., V. S. entire	1	39	Birth			1				1				1			1		1				1	1				
	(b) A. from both ventricles.	7	48	15m	25	3	3		2	7	5		2	3	7			2	3	2	6	6	3	7	4	4			1
	(c) A. from R. V.	3	13m	13w	10m	1		1		3	1				3							3		1					
	(d) A. from R. V., double conus.	1					1	1	1	1	1			1	1						1	1			1	1			
	2. Complete transposition:																												
	(a) Closed V. S.	32	11	2d	6m	16	4	23	30		5		4	3	32				1	2	12	23	3	4	9	13			
	(b) Defect V. S.	17	16	6d	2¾	11	3	10	14	17	7	7	2	1	16	1			1	2	6	10		3	10	8	3		
	3. Partial transposition.	16	20	12d	4½	8	5	6	10	16	3	10	4	2	11					4	6	8	1	6	16	13	3		
	4. Corrected transposition.	4	24	9w	11¼	3	1		1	4	2	1		1				1	1		1	3		3	4	3			

Series numbers	Classification of Defects	Clinical: History: Hereditary predisposition	Personal: Rheumatism	Tuberculosis	Congenital syphilis	Infec. dis., recovery	Cyanosis: Slight	Moderate	Marked	Terminal	Clubbing	Dyspnea	Dyspneic attacks	Syncopic attacks	Delayed development	Polycythemia	Cardiac: Precordial bulging	Pulsation	Thrill: Systolic	Diastolic, early, late	Continuous, double	Dulness + above	Second sound +	Murmurs: Systolic	Diastolic	Presystolic	Double	Continuous
I	**Anomalies of pericardium:**																											
	1. Pericardial defects.		1	5		1						2					1		1				1	1				
	2. Diverticulum.																											
II	**Displacements of the heart:**																											
	1. Ectopia cordis.	2			1					2														1				
	2. "Isolated" Dextrocardia																											
	(a) Without inversion chambers	1		1		1	2	1	4		3	5	2	1	3	2	1		2			2	2	6				
	(b) With inversion chambers.	2				2		1	6		4	6	3		4	1	1	2				1	2	2				
	3. Dextrocardia with situs inversus.	1						1	6		2	1			1		1	1					2	3				
	4. Incomplete heterotaxy.	2				1	1	3	1		1	2	1		2	1			1			1		3				
	5. Dextroposition cordis.					1			1		1	2					1	2						1				
III	**Anomalies of the heart as a whole:**																											
	1. Bifid apex.																											
	2. Diverticulum.				1																							
	3. Primary congenital hypertrophy.	3					2	1		4		7	3	4	1		3					1	2	6				
	4. Congenital rhabdomyoma.					3				1				1	6									2				
	5. Congenital heart block.	1		1					3		2	1			1	2	1		1				1	3	1			
IV	**Anomalous septa or chordæ:**																											
	1. Anomalous septa (a) in L. A.	1				1			2	1		5	1		1	1		1					1	4		1		
	(b) in R. A.			1																								
	(c) in ventricles.	1				1			3		2	1	2		1			1		1				2				
	2. Anomalous chordæ (a) in L. A.			1		1																	1	1				
	(b) in R. A.																											
	(c) in ventricles.		1								1							1	2	1			3				2	
	(d) in aorta.																											
V	**Defects of interauricular septum:**																											
	1. Patent foramen ovale.	7	4	2		3	4	3	1	21	2	21	6		12		6	7	2	4		6	8	11	1	10	1	
	2. Defects auricular septum above.	1								3		3		1						1		1	1	2		2		
	3. Defects auricular septum below.	2	4	1		2	1			7		5	1		5	1	3	5	3	1	2	1	4	6	2	3	1	
	4. Multiple defects, auricular septum.		1							1		2							1					2	1			
	5. Premature closure F. O.								2																			
VI	**Defects of interventricular septum:**																											
	1. At base (a) without dextroposition.	3	3	6	1	12	3		1	12	1	14	3	1	4		5	4	19			3	2	38			3	1
	2. Defects elsewhere or multiple.			1				1		1			1		1				2					3				
	3. Aneurysms of pars membranacea.			2													1	1	1				1	2				
VII	**Complete defects of cardiac septa:**																											
	1. Cor triloculare biventriculare.							4			1	3				1			1					2				
	2. Cor triloculare biatriatum.	2					3	3	3	2	1	6	5		1	1								5				1
	3. Cor biloculare.	1		1		1	1	3	4		1	3	2		1			1										1
	4. Incomplete double heart.	2		1				2	1	4	1	4	3		6	2		3	1					6				
VIII	**Defects of aortic septum:**																											
	1. Persistent truncus (complete defect).	3	1	1				3	10	1	5	7	6		3	3	1	2	2	2			2	5	2	1	1	
	2. Communication between A. and P. A.	1		2		4				4		3					2	1	1				1	2			3	
	3. Congen. aneur. of right aortic sinus.		3	1		1		1		4		7					1	2	1	1	3	1	4				4	5
IX	**Transposition of arterial trunks:**																											
	1. Dextroposition of aorta.																											
	(a) A. from L. V., V. S. entire	1				1																						
	(b) A. from both ventricles.						1	1	2	2	2	5				1		1	2		1	1		3		3		
	(c) A. from R. V.						1		2				1		2		2							3				
	(d) A. from R. V., double conus.																											
	2. Complete transposition:																											
	(a) Closed V. S.	3			1	1	1	5	16		4	9	11			1	3	5				2	1	8				
	(b) Defect V. S.	4				1		3	13	1	5	6	3		3	2	1	2	3				2	10			1	
	3. Partial transposition.	1		3		1	1	3	4	2	4	4	2		3	2	2	4	1			2	3	5		1	1	
	4. Corrected transposition.																1		1				2	1			1	

Series numbers	Classification of Defects	Causes of Death: Cardio-vasc. Defect: Sudden	Cardiac insufficiency	Stillborn	Bronchopneumonia	Cerebral disease	Bacterial endocarditis or endarteritis	Other causes	Relative Frequency: Number classified as primary lesion	Number complicating other defects	Total incidence
I	**Anomalies of pericardium:**										
	1. Pericardial defects.	1	6	2	1	2		13	30	1	**31**
	2. Diverticulum.		3						6		**6**
II	**Displacements of the heart:**										
	1. Ectopia cordis.			4	1			1	7	1	**8**
	2. "Isolated" Dextrocardia										
	(a) Without inversion chambers	2	1		1			3	8	5	**13**
	(b) With inversion chambers.	5	4	1	1				10	1	**11**
	3. Dextrocardia with situs inversus.	4	4	2	1				11	4	**15**
	4. Incomplete heterotaxy.	1			2			1	5	3	**8**
	5. Dextroposition cordis.		2					1	3	1	**4**
III	**Anomalies of the heart as a whole:**										
	1. Bifid apex.								4	15	**19**
	2. Diverticulum.			1	1				3	1	**4**
	3. Primary congenital hypertrophy.	5	4	1	3	1			15	2	**17**
	4. Congenital rhabdomyoma.	7	2	2		1		5	17		**17**
	5. Congenital heart block.	3							3	1	**4**
IV	**Anomalous septa or chordæ:**										
	1. Anomalous septa (a) in L. A.		2	1	2			2	10	3	**13**
	(b) in R. A.						2		4	13	**17**
	(c) in ventricles.	2	1						3	10	**13**
	2. Anomalous chordæ (a) in L. A.		1		1		1	1	7	4	**11**
	(b) in R. A.	3	2						5	13	**18**
	(c) in ventricles.							6	6	5	**11**
	(d) in aorta.				2			2	5	1	**6**
V	**Defects of interauricular septum:**										
	1. Patent foramen ovale.	7	18		2	2		7	40	250	**290**
	2. Defects auricular septum above.	1	5					2	10	9	**19**
	3. Defects auricular septum below.		7		4		2	2	18	18	**36**
	4. Multiple defects, auricular septum.		2			1		2	5	23	**28**
	5. Premature closure F. O.		1	1		1			3	1	**4**
VI	**Defects of interventricular septum:**										
	1. At base (a) without dextroposition.	4	4	1	10	3	13	16	50	207	**257**
	2. Defects elsewhere or multiple.	1				1		1	5	12	**17**
	3. Aneurysms of pars membranacea.				1			6	7	9	**16**
VII	**Complete defects of cardiac septa:**										
	1. Cor triloculare biventriculare.		5						5	10	**15**
	2. Cor triloculare biatriatum.	4	4	1			2		13	14	**27**
	3. Cor biloculare.	3	2			1		1	9	5	**14**
	4. Incomplete double heart.	2	3		2			2	10	4	**14**
VIII	**Defects of aortic septum:**										
	1. Persistent truncus (complete defect).	2	7	3	1		1	3	21	13	**34**
	2. Communication between A. and P. A.	1	4					2	10		**10**
	3. Congen. aneur. of right aortic sinus.	1	9				2		12		**12**
IX	**Transposition of arterial trunks:**										
	1. Dextroposition of aorta.										
	(a) A. from L. V., V. S. entire							1	1	1	**2**
	(b) A. from both ventricles.		2		1	1	2	1	7	63	**70**
	(c) A. from R. V.		1						3	48	**51**
	(d) A. from R. V., double conus.			1					1	1	**2**
	2. Complete transposition:										
	(a) Closed V. S.	12	4		1	2		1	32	6	**38**
	(b) Defect V. S.	4	3		4	1		1	17	19	**36**
	3. Partial transposition.	2	3			2		2	16	15	**31**
	4. Corrected transposition.	1	3		1				4	2	**6**

X Pulmonary stenosis:
1. With closed septa.
2. With patent F. O. closed V. S.
3. With closed F. O. defect V. S.
4. With patent F. O. and defect V. S.

XI Pulmonary atresia:
1. With closed V. S.
2. With closed F. O., defect V. S.
3. With patent F. O., defect V. S.

XII Pulmonary insufficiency or dilatation:
1. Valvular insufficiency
2. Congenital dilatation P. A.

XIII Aortic stenosis and atresia:
1. Subaortic stenosis.
2. Aortic stenosis.
3. Aortic atresia.

XIV Anomalies of semilunar cusps:
1. Supernumerary cusps (a) of P. V.
                  (b) of A. V.
2. Reduced no. (a) Bicuspid P. V.
             (b) Bicuspid A. V.
3. Defect (a) of P. V.
        (b) of A. V.

XV Tricuspid and mitral stenoses:
1. Tricuspid stenosis.
2. Tricuspid atresia.
3. Mitral stenosis.
4. Mitral atresia.

XVI Anomalies of a-v cusps:
1. Double orifices (a) of T. O.
                (b) of M. O.
2. Insuff. or defect (a) of T. V.
                 (b) of M. V.

XVII Patent ductus arteriosus:
1. Simple patency.
2. So-called aneurysm.
3. Absence of D. A.

XVIII Coarctation of the aorta:
1. Adult type.
2. Infantile type.
3. P. A. forms descending aorta.

XIX Hypoplasia of the aorta.

XX Anomalies of aortic arch:
1. Double aortic arch.
2. Right aortic arch.
3. Absence aortic arch.
4. Rt. subclavian from desc. A.
5. Lt. subclavian from D. A. or P. A.
6. Common brachioceph. trunk

XXI Anomalous coronaries:
1. Origin from P. A.
2. Rt. cor. into cor. sinus
3. Aneurysm rt. coronary.

XXII Anomalous pulmonary arteries.

XXIII Anomalies of great veins:
1. Of systemic V. (persist. L. S. V. C.).
2. Of pulmonary veins.

XXIV Congenital arteriovenous aneurysm.

Abbreviations: A = Aorta   P. A. = Pulmonary artery   V. S. = Interventricular septum   A. S. = Interauricular septum   D. A. = Ductus arteriosus   F. O. = Foramen ovale

a-v = auriculo-ventricular   h = hours   d = days   w = weeks   m = months

INDEX